Why You Get Sick and How Your Brain Can Fix It!

Richard G. Barwell, DC

Foreward by Patrick K. Porter, Ph.D.
Author of "Thrive In Overdrive,
How to Navigate Your Overloaded Lifestyle"

Richard G. Barwell, DC
NeuroInfiniti
#503 - 188 Pinellas Lane,
Cocoa Beach, Florida,32931
Phone: 321 868 5690
Email:drbarwell@neuroInifiniti.com
Website: www.NeuroInfiniti.com

Disclaimer: This book is designed to provide information in regard to the subject matter covered. It is sold with the understanding that the publisher and author are not engaged in rendering medical advice. The information in this book is non-diagnostic and is not intended to replace medical treatment. If medical or other expert assistance is required, the services of a licensed professional should be sought. The purpose of this book is to educate and entertain. The publisher, author, or any dealer or distributor shall not be liable to the purchaser or any other person or entity with respect to any liability, loss, or damage caused or alleged to be caused directly or indirectly by this book. **If you do not wish to be bound by the above, you may return this book for a full refund.**

First Edition: Aug 2013

ISBN:1-4392-2207-X

Printed in the United States of America

TABLE OF CONTENTS

###

"Today's challenges and crises in healthcare emphasize the need for a fundamental paradigm shift in the conventional healing arts. Why You Get Sick ..., Richard G. Barwell, DC's readable synthesis of frontier science and professional experience, is a significant contribution in helping the public move beyond misperceived limitations and write new empowering stories for themselves. Richard's insights, illuminating the connections among mind, nervous and immune systems, reveal how stress unconsciously sabotages our health, and how, with an "informed" consciousness, we can exercise mastery over our biology. The knowledge in this book is profoundly self-empowering. "

Bruce H. Lipton, Ph.D., Cell biologist and bestselling author of The Biology of Belief: Unleashing the Power of Consciousness, Matter and Miracles and his most recent book, The Honeymoon Effect: The Science of Creating Heaven on Earth

###

Acknowledgements

This is the page which every author adds to their book knowing that it will only be read by a few. Since being involved in the effort required to bring a book to life I have found myself reading the "thank you" pages of others from start to finish. This book represents a journey - a lifetime journey that wasn't accomplished alone. It starts with my parents who gave me the freedom to make decisions, but also taught me that I had to take responsibility for those decisions. My decision to enter Chiropractic carried with it the responsibility to strive for the highest level of excellence throughout my career. I had the good fortune to have instructors such as Drs. Homewood, Hines and Watkins during my time at Canadian Memorial Chiropractic College, who taught more than just book-based information.

I had the opportunity to pick mentors such as Drs. Joe Flesia and Guy Riekeman, who coached me through many challenges and kept me searching for a better understanding of the power of chiropractic. To Drs. Annette Long and her husband Dr. Alvah Byers I will always owe a debt of gratitude. Through their guidance and joint effort we uncovered the direct brain connection which opened the door to finding the missing link for the Chiropractic profession.

Dr. Doug Meints has been pushing me to write this book for about 14 years so here it is Dr. Doug! Thanks for the PUSH. (Otherwise known as nag, nag). Dr. Doug's nagging has been followed by further pushes from David and DeDe Van Riper and Carriann Terzini, who are a critical part of the NeuroInfiniti team.

While Dr. Patrick Porter was the one who provided the wherewithal to actually bring this book to reality, it is to two ladies that I owe most of the credit. Dr. Cynthia Porter took control of the final steps and finished bringing my dream to life. Many thanks to Cynthia for the great detail work.

My deepest gratitude and largest thanks must go to my wonderful wife Susan, who has been my inspiration and partner throughout my years of growth, discontent, and shifts in practice. Susan has had the terrible task of editing my writing, spelling and crazy run on and on and on sentence structure.

I will close this with my mantra:

My God lives in me and through me; I may die today; I need to take care of others; and we are all equal.

May this book bring you to health and happiness.

RGB

Foreword

When I met Dr. Barwell and his staff in 2008, I was immediately captivated by his philosophy on health, healing and chiropractic, and by the connections he had made between psychology, neurology and physiology. It was a conversation no one else was having; yet the implications of his research, and the related neurological tools he had developed, were nothing short of a monumental shift in how healthcare could and should be delivered in our fast-paced, over-stressed world.

Over the last two and a half decades, I have trained and worked with hundreds of chiropractic physicians and have been introduced to equally as many tools and techniques of the trade, but in all that time, I had never come across another integrated approach that brought together the foundational tools of neurology—neurofeedback and chiropractic care—to achieve unparalleled results for today's most pressing problems.

As my relationship with Dr. Barwell grew, and when he later invited me to attend his training events, I was able to learn more about the amazing breakthroughs he and his team of doctors all over the world were getting as a matter of course, and the results are nothing short of astounding. Within these pages you'll read a variety of stories and testimonials that demonstrate just how powerful this neurological training can be.

Today, Dr. Barwell has made revitalizing chiropractic care his mission, and he's doing just that by bringing chiropractic full circle—back to its roots in neurology. What you have in your hands is just the tip of the iceberg in relation to his research and breakthrough systems, but that doesn't mean you should take this book lightly. Rather, look upon it as the groundbreaking achievement it is—a work I predict will one day be looked upon as the dawn of the early 21st Century medical revolution. I feel confident in saying this because Dr. Barwell has already left his mark on the field, and with the help of readers like you who seek and share breakthroughs like this, his mission of having neurologically-based chiropractic available in every city around the world will become a reality. In fact, he has already put together a team from around the globe that is validating his work every day.

If you are a chiropractor, you will learn a new language; a way to change the conversation with your patients and colleagues. You will discover, just as other NeuroInfiniti Doctors have, that the time is now for the world to say no more! to sickness-based healthcare and to usher in the new era of neurologically-based wellness with holistic-minded chiropractic physicians leading the way. If you get a chance to sit in or listen to one of Dr. Barwell's talks about this topic, you will realize that you owe it to yourself to rediscover neurologically-based chiropractic for yourself. You will want to research these tools and then invest in the knowledge and technology, so that you, too, can be a part of this movement that is creating vibrant good health for so many patients.

If you are an end user or patient at one of the hundreds of clinics using Neuro-Infiniti technology, you will get a look behind the curtain into the realm of neurology and brain science. You will gain a better understanding of the powerful connection between your thoughts, actions and beliefs and your health. You'll also come to see how correct chiropractic care is the best and brightest solution for reversing our current health crisis.

Before you get started, I want to remind you to read the collection of success stories found within these pages to help you better understand how neurologically-based chiropractic is transforming lives. Later, we would love to hear about your results and how learning about the brain/body connection and brain wave entrainment has improved the quality of your life.

My wish for you is to read this text with an open mind. Your current beliefs about wellness and chiropractic might be challenged, but as Dr. Barwell weaves together real-life stories and science, you will come to understand the promise of this breakthrough and will want to discover it for yourself. I'm confident you'll be as enthralled with Dr. Barwell's discoveries as I am and as excited as the thousands of successful patients who are using this technology to create optimum health every day.

Yours in health,

Patrick K. Porter, Ph.D.
Author of "Thrive in Overdrive, How to Navigate Your Overloaded Lifestyle"

Introduction

On this particular day in 1974, after 10 years of chiropractic practice experience, I had no idea that my introduction to a child named "Kim" would begin my lifetime search for truth. When Kim's mother came into the office for care, she brought along her 3 year old daughter, Kim. She placed Kim on the floor and I addressed the mother's challenges, but there was something about Kim that kept my attention. I noted there wasn't any movement or sounds coming from Kim, and asked her mother to tell me Kim's story.

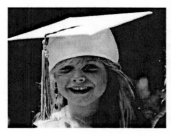

The story revealed that Kim had been born with the umbilical cord wrapped around her neck and she had suffered brain damage. In the three years of this child's life, there had been no responses, no movement, no sound, and no recognition of anything. Kim was basically in a catatonic state.

Her parents had taken Kim to every specialist possible and were told that this was simply the way Kim was and nothing was ever going to change. By this day in 1974, the parents had resolved themselves to Kim's condition and just did their best to cope.

I asked the mother if I could examine Kim and she said agreed. The first thing I noted was that no matter what I did, such as holding her, moving her, or creating movement in front of her eyes, there was absolutely no sign of response. There was no acknowledgement of awareness, period.

The next thing I noted was that there was an odd shape to her head. I traced the joints of the skull and found some irregular patterns. I applied some gentle directional pressure and asked to have Kim brought in each time with the mother. On the third visit something strange happened. As I applied the pressure, Kim made a sound! It was just a little "Uhh," but it was something.

It was interesting but we thought it was just coincidence. On the next visit she did it again. This was the first time she had reacted to anything in her life, and by the sixth visit, she made the sound before I touched her. By the next visit, she made the sound when she saw me. Something big was happening in all of our lives. Then she started putting her own hands on her head when she saw me. I continued to see Kim over the next few years and watched her develop into a healthy active girl with a wonderful sense of humor. The last time I saw Kim she was 21 years old, had a job and a future. The story doesn't end there!

While the reward to Kim and her family is obvious, my reward goes far beyond the gratification of my role in this wonderful experience. It led me to look at chiropractic and a question I had never before considered. I didn't follow the typical chiropractic protocol of correcting vertebral subluxation (so-called misaligned vertebra) yet I saw the dramatic changes in Kim's life. How could this be? Was chiropractic something beyond moving bones of the spine? It must have been, because Kim's response had nothing to do with spinal joint correction. Everything I had been taught at chiropractic college was based on abnormal joint position of the spine and correction. Something else was at play and thanks to the Kim experience, my life had a bigger mission. I needed to find out why Kim came to life with something as simple as some skull molding.

Here was a child given no hope by modern medicine. She had no infections and adding drugs to her life would have only made matters worse. The chiropractic technique I used was outside the typical concepts of chiropractic, yet here was the incredible result of a normal human being. There had to be more to the story of what not only defines health but also something beyond the model of treating people only for pain relief, whether through medicine, or regular chiropractic. What follows in the book is a guide through my thirty-year search to understand what happened to Kim and the thousands of others throughout the years, who have had their lives changed by healing approaches that make no sense within the boundaries of drug-based medicine or spinal correction chiropractic.

This book is about a journey and I hope you find it as rewarding as I have, traveling the path to a new understanding of life and health. Some parts of the path may be steeper than others, but stay with it and in the end you will find the destination empowering.

CHAPTER
ONE

The Intent of this book

Chapter 1

The Intent of this book

The intent of this book is to expose failings in our health services and to present information needed to change the direction of the health care system. The book is written for both the public and the keepers of the system. The current so-called "Health Care System" has disempowered the individual through education that has convinced him/her into thinking that modern medicine not only has all the answers, but also is scientifically based. Both of these beliefs are false! While medicine has made great strides in lifesaving events such as heart, liver and other transplants, the basic medical practice has fallen under the control of Wall Street and Big Pharma[1,2]. Together they are responsible for the "Sickness Care System" in which care takes place only after you have become ill. Today there is a new field emerging and it is coming from neuroscience research. This research into brain function and its relationship to health and disease is painting a new picture for all. Our ability to adapt, to respond to and recover from stress, has been elevated to a central role in our ability to remain healthy as well as in the creation of disease.

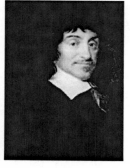

"I think, therefore I am…" Rene Descartes. The significance of this statement is that it really brings the role of brain function into perspective. The power of thought, whether conscious or subconscious, creates your perception of the world around you and controls your ability to respond to it. The seat of consciousness lies within the brain; and so I thought this was rather fitting to say *I think, therefore I am"*. But, we need to understand what

---

1   Insider Report on Big Pharma's Corrupt Marketing and Phony Science - Topics: Dubious statistics, Health care, Regulations and regulators, Science and the scientific method - http://www.naked-capitalism.com/2012/07/insider-reports-on-big-pharmas-corrupt-marketing-and-phony-science.html#j7jyUvCsuw8T9FHs.99

2   Big Pharma's Bitter Pill by Joe Mantone - The Wall Street Journal news - Wednesday, September 12, 2012 As of 4:56 PM EDT

"I think" implies and entails.

The Descartes' statement of "*I think, therefore I am,.*" is somewhat lacking when we consider the effects of today's strife and stressors in our life. Perhaps a more appropriate statement would be, "*I think, so maybe I am not.*" This book will present a better understanding of all that "*I think*" implies in the role of disease and/or health.

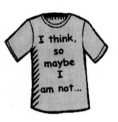

The current study of the relationship between thought, brain function and stress has found a new perspective on the meaning of disease and/or health. Our Central Nervous System (CNS), the seat of thought, can short circuit as a result of stress overload and create patterns of disruption in neurological function. Research has discovered that these patterns of thought processes are producing inappropriate physical responses[3]. The outcome of these inappropriate responses creates physical stressors, which in turn create signs and symptoms. These signs and symptoms are the foundation of all disease. So do you have a disease or just a damaged series of neurological processes that have been named as a disease? The current research tells us the latter is the real problem. We need to be looking at *why* the CNS is malfunctioning and creating the confusion, misdirection and inappropriate responses which lead to the development of all so called disease.

Welcome to the world of Neuroscience!

If the last paragraph has you already feeling uncomfortable with the direction of this book, good! It simply means that you have realized that what you have been taught, as opposed to what you just read, has put you on the defensive. I see that same reaction each time I speak, whether it is to my own profession or an outside group. We continually look to our educational history for verification of our beliefs be-

3   Brain Economics: - Housekeeping Routines in the Brain   - Proefschriftterverkrijging van het doctoraat in de MedischeWetenschappenaan de Rijksuniversiteit Groningen op gezag van de Rector Magnificus, dr. F. Zwarts, in het openbaarteverdedigen op maandag 5 oktober 2009 om 14.45 uur door Paolo Toffaningeboren op 12 maart 1979 teSandrigo, Itali"ePromotores : Prof. dr. A. Johnson Prof. dr. R. de Jong Prof. dr. G.J. ter Horst Copromotor : Dr. S. Martens Beoordelingscommissie : Prof. dr. M. Eimer Prof. dr. B. Hommel Prof. dr. N.M. Maurits ISBN (boek): 978-90-367-3979-5 ISBN (digitaal): 978-90-367-3978-8

cause that is where those beliefs were developed. What most fail to recognize is that the institutions of education are anchored in the past. New concepts and directions may come out of the research done at the post graduate level, but they are seldom received with joy or in a timely manner within the course programs of the universities. Then we have to consider the practicing health practitioners, among whom new graduates, with new ideas, are looked upon as upstarts. The one area of new concepts or product introduction that is met with easy approval is pharmaceutical, with their promises of magical properties and their short cuts to health. Just watch the TV ads, but be sure to listen to the possibility of developing all those nasty effects. It is past time for the truth to be told and for the public to learn about better choices in their health future.

A paper on *Cause of Disease: A New Perspective*[4]"outlines how the latest research on neurological function, changes the model of health care. Medical, dental and chiropractic views are all changing as a result of new information regarding the cause of disease and illness.

Today we know that the old medical concepts of the germ theory are no longer valid and that stress is playing a much more important role in directly affecting general health. We now know that the old medical concept regarding the immune system as a stand-alone system in the body was wrong and that Psychoneuroimmunology[5] is the key to understanding the body's resistance to disease. With these revelations comes the need for all health professions to revisit their position, dialog, definitions and intent of care.

When the world went from horses to motor cars for transportation, it not only changed the mode of travel but also the dialog and procedures involved. Feed bags and grooming just did not apply to the new world of cars. When we consider the medical germ theory[6] and/

---

4   A White PaperCause of Disease : A New PerspectiveBy Richard Barwell, DC

5   Latest Research Reveals Stress Factors Outweigh Germs as Cause of Disease. Published The Chiropractic Journal Volume   Research pointing to a circuit linking the immune system and brain connects illness, stress, mood and thought in a whole new way. By BETH AZAR   American Psychological Association - December 2001, Vol. 32, No. 11   Print version: page 34

6   The germ theory of disease, also called the pathogenic theory of medicine, is a theory that proposes that microorganisms are the cause of many diseases. Although highly controversial when first proposed, it is now a cornerstone of modern medicine and clinical microbiology, leading to such important innovations as antibiotics and hygienic practices.[1]

or chiropractic's spinal nerve root pressure theory[7]" as compared to psychoneuroimmunology and compromised neural integrity (CNI)", the leap is as great as from horses to motor cars. The new science has changed not only the rules but also the game and the dialog as well. It is therefore appropriate to visit the historical viewpoints of these two professions.

Chapter 1 - Things to Consider

☞ Do you consider Kim's story just a story, or do you see the potential in understanding what happened?

☞ What is the relevance in "I think" regarding current models of health care?

☞ Are you aware of the connection between medicine and "Wall Street"?

☞ Have you ever wondered about the cause of disease?

☞ Have you ever wondered about why some people get sick while others don't?

☞ Do you think you have a role in your health future?

☞ Do you listen to the TV ads for drugs sales - including the dangers of taking them?

---

7   "Subluxation is a complex of functional and/or structural and/or pathological articular changes that compromise neural integrity and may influence organ system function and general health". J Can ChioprAssoc 2002; 46(4) 215 EF Owens * Director of Research - Sherman College of Straight Chiropractic

Absolute Angel

How important is it for a 9 year old girl to have a sleep over? I have been treating a young girl with such severe anxiety that she was not able to have a sleep over with her friends; either her house or another's house. We have done three months of chiropractic and neurofeedback and the mom reported to me that her behavior has improved so much that they celebrated last weekend by allowing her to invite two of her friends over for a sleep over. The mom reported that she "was an absolute angel" and had an awesome night with her friends!!

Ralph Cardin, DC
Provider of Neurologically-based Chiropractic
Overland Park KS, USA
drralph@cardinwellness.com

CHAPTER
TWO

The Law of the Lie:
The Germ Is Not
the Cause of Disease.

Chapter 2

The Law of the Lie:

The "Germ Theory" is Not the Cause of Disease

Chiropractic and medicine are different in both their application and philosophical construct. Medical philosophy follows the construct of *reductionism* or *mechanism*[1]. This philosophy holds that if you
can study the parts and replace the damaged part, the whole will work
right. Chiropractic follows the philosophy of *vitalism*. The vitalistic
philosophy[2] holds that the sum is greater than its parts and that there is
an element of vital force of life beyond the parts. You cannot use terms
or applications of an orange when discussing an apple. This is not just
a game of semantics.

It is important at this point to demonstrate some of the basic differences between the medical model and the chiropractic model of health
concepts. The terms *diagnosis* and *treatment* are used in the definition
of the practice of medicine. The term diagnosis comes from the historical background of medicine. This explanation is not meant to belittle
medicine but rather to show how the term has become so important. It
starts with the medicine man or healers of the past, during which time
people who were sick were thought to have been possessed by some
spirit. The role of the healer was to identify the spirit and develop a
treatment that would rid the body of the spirit or entity. This concept
still exists today in medicine. Signs and symptoms are grouped together and given the name of a disease, which is then called a diagnosis. A
treatment is then prescribed with the intent to rid the body of the disease. A disease is then treated as an entity and current terminology supports this -such as "I **caught** a cold" or "I **have** cancer." We have just
moved the concept of illness being an entity or bad spirit to a symptom

---

1   ReductionismRandom House Dictionary, © Random House, Inc. 2010. re·duc·tion·ism - noun 1. the theory
    that every complex phenomenon, esp. in biology or psychology, can be explained by analyzing the simplest,
    most basic physical mechanisms that are in operation during the phenomenon. 2. the practice of simplifying
    a complex idea, issue, condition, or the like, esp. to the point of minimizing, obscuring, or distorting it. Origin:
    1940–45; reductionism

2   VitalismJonas: Mosby's Dictionary of Complementary and Alternative Medicine. (c) 2005, Elsevier. - vitalismn
    doctrine that a nonphysical energy permeates all living organisms and that gives them the property of life.

group and called it disease. The greatest challenge to this approach is that one has to wait until the signs and symptoms appear before any treatment can be applied. This time delay removes modern medicine from a field of *health generation* to a profession of *disease management*.

Then along came the germ theory[3]. That made it very simple for the medical field. The medical profession said, now we know the cause of disease. We know it is these bacteria, or germs, that are causing our ill health. Their next step was to make chemicals (called antibiotics) that kill all the germs! Outside of the fact that this move has now created a world of super-germs", the real cause wasn't the germs after all. Germs (bacteria and viruses) have been around since before humans and they outnumber humans. So how is it that some people are in the same room as a flu virus, but only some of them "get it" and some of them don't? If the cause of the flu was the virus, and it was present, then they should all get it. This is not what happens. Even when the medical researchers knew that this question was in play, rather than deal with this inconsistency in the germ theory it was easier to just treat the symptoms, so pharmaceutical companies devised treatments (medicines/drugs) to kill bacteria and to reduce the symptoms.

Therefore, the relationship between the medical profession and drug companies was born and those two worked together to form one of the largest, most powerful lobbies ever. In the past three decades, America's healthcare system has radically metamorphosed from a public service network (largely run by independent physicians and nonprofit hospitals) into a corporate profit machine-one that Dr. Arnold Relman, the renowned former editor of the *New England Journal of Medicine*, calls the Medical-industrial Complex.[4] The problem is that the germ theory today is dead. It no longer exists. Why? Because neuroscience has a better explanation for the loss of ideal health.

This doesn't mean there aren't bacteria or viruses out there. Abso-

---

3   The germ theory of disease, also called the pathogenic theory of medicine, is a theory that proposes that microorganisms are the cause of many diseases. Although highly controversial when first proposed, it is now a cornerstone of modern medicine and clinical microbiology, leading to such important innovations as antibiotics and hygienic practices.

4   How The Profit-Hungry "Medical-Industrial Complex" Hurts Health Care (VIDEO) Bill Moyers - Huffingtion PostFirst Posted: 09/28/09 06:12 AM ETUpdated: 05/25/11 02:55 PM ET

lutely not! What has been revealed is that being healthy has to do with the body's ability to deal with the viruses and bacteria. It means that we are now looking at how to make the body strong enough to resist those critters rather than trying to kill them once they have invaded the body.

The introduction of penicillin, the wonder drug of the 1940s, lulled the world into a false sense of security when it came to health. Problems with antibiotic therapy arose very quickly. Even the discoverer of penicillin warned that we should not be over doing this. We began only using a few units and now we have to use a million units for the same infection. Our germ phobia world, especially in North America, has gotten to the point where it has created super-bugs through overuse of antibiotics. Bacteria are living things which have learned to adapt and, in fact, some have turned the antibiotics into food. These super-bugs are getting stronger[5] and more numerous to the point where there is no defense whatsoever from some of them. We are seeing a resurgence in diseases such as tuberculosis, along with some very nasty bacteria such as the one that creates the "flesh eating disease" (MRSA) and a new one that produces non-curable pneumonia (klebsiellapneumoniae). That old system has broken down, and the problem is that the medical doctors know it and are caught by their own marketing. They don't want to just hand out antibiotics, but now the patients are demanding them. Rather than putting up with a screaming parent who wants an antibiotic for their child, they give it to them. I don't blame them, because having a screaming parent demanding, "Do something for my child," is not a pleasant situation. This challenge of restricting prescriptions has placed the medical doctor in a very precarious position, to the point where an article was published in one of the leading medical journals on the impact of the end of antibiotics—The article indicated that the growth of antibiotic use was the most effective therapy in medical history; however,the collapse of antibiotic therapy represents the downfall of the medical cultural authority leaving them with an alternative of "Act like you care," and suggesting that MDs take acting lessons.[6] It's

5   Antibiotic Resistance: The 5 Riskiest Superbugs - By Katie MoisseMarch 27, 2012   ABC NEWS.com

6   Acting in medical practice. Conter D, Finestone H, MD.The Lancet.1994;344:801-2.

time for us as a society to stop buying into this old germ theory and start looking at the other concepts of how to be healthy. We should be improving our immune systems rather than trying to kill the bacteria or treat the symptoms.

History reveals that the great advancement in health lies in the development of improved public health[7]. Sanitary sewage systems, improved food storage, the invention of soap, clean safe water supplies and the increase in the public's education with regard to this issue were more important than the development of antibiotics. The plagues of the past were not created by the lack of medicine. Now we are looking at the role of factors such as mass transit, overcrowding, airline transmission of bacteria and viruses to which our systems have not had the opportunity to develop our natural immunity, as health threats. The exposure to these viruses and bacteria run a course then die out.[8] The reason is that our systems are able to adapt and build antibodies to counter the invaders. Every challenge to our health has been met with an immune response that ensures the human race of survival. The cost is high, for thousands may die, but hundreds adapt and live. Those hundreds pass on the ability to survive through our innate immune responses

Chapter 2 - Things to Consider

☞ Were you aware of the two basic philosophies in health care?

☞ Do you understand these philosophies establish who has control over your health?

☞ Which approach do you think has the greatest benefit – relying on drugs to maintain health, or strengthening your body's natural systems to provide protection?

☞ Are you aware that vaccinations came into play after the natural

---

7   The Population Health Approach in Historical Perspective - Am J Public Health. 2003 March; 93(3): 421–431. PMCID: PMC1449802 - Simon Szreter, PhD

8   A Shot in the Dark (Paperback) by Harris L. Coulter and Barbara Loe Fisher

immune system had already lessened the effects of the disease? (In every case)?

☞ The "germ theory" failed to offer any explanation as to how some people were resistant to a germ.

☞ Did you know that Alexander Flemming warned medicine not to over use penicillin?

☞ Have you ever wondered why diseases such as: SARS, Ebola, AIDS, and Swine FLU start and stop?

The Daffodils

At a revolutionary seminar with Dr. Richard Barwell I heard," we are called to be Chiropractors." That's true for me because I resisted becoming a Chiropractor for as long as I could. When I surrendered and went to Life Chiropractic University I then became one of the few fourth generation Chiropractors of my time.

Throughout my 32 year journey I have had the great privilege of being a part of so many exciting and unexpected miracles. One of the experiences that stands out for me is with Joe B. I was in my office when I got a call from Grady Hospital in Atlanta. The nurse was calling in family and friends to see Joe whom they said was dying of Aids. I went that day to see him and have my last connection, to let him know I loved him. When I walked into the hospital room I saw Joe hooked up to all kinds of wires. When he saw me he could barely mumble a hello. I did my best to comfort him and send all of my love to him. When it was time for me to go I asked him if he would like me to adjust his atlas, the first bone in the neck that is neurologically rich and provides enormous input to the brain. No matter what someone's physical state is, I feel like it's a blessing to receive a Chiropractic Adjustment. He simply nodded. I moved behind the bed, adjusted him and said, "The power's on!" It's what I say after giving most of my adjustments. It means that the innate power of the body is now flowing. It felt good to give him that gift. Yet I was drowning in the sadness for the loss of a 19 year old extraordinarily talented and wonderful person. After I left the room I ran back in and said, "See you tomorrow Joe." This whole experience weighed heavy on my heart. The next day determined to see him again I went back. He was still alive and on leaving I adjusted him again. The next day I went and he was sitting up in his room, laughing and talking with the nurses. The same story again. The next day when I showed up he was walking down the hall rolling the fluid bags and talking to everyone who passed. He had the joy of being alive vibrating from him. One more visit and adjustment and then the Doctors were saying, Well we don't understand this but Joe can go home tomorrow. They didn't understand, but I did. I know to never underestimate the power of a Chiropractic Adjustment. I have seen so many miracles in my lifetime.

Now the new problem was, he didn't have any place to go home to. Mary Ann and I talked and we agreed Joe could come to our home and recover. For the next year Joe lived with us. Throughout the first three months he spent most of his days lying on the couch barely talking. When he would eat he would have to run to the bathroom to throw up or have explosive diarrhea. He really struggled with his health. Some days I would come home from the office and Joe's temperature would be so high that he was drenched in sweat. I would adjust him and his fever would break and he would sleep peacefully. With adjustments the body's immune system is strengthened and then the body does its best to go into balance. The high fevers had worked in his favor to help his body to heal. We continued on, giving an adjustment every day. Joe was adamant he was not going to the medical doctor, that if he was going to die he would do that peacefully at home, our home.

The year was up and down, but delightfully Joe was getting stronger and stronger. His life force was increasing and his hopes, dreams, and talents were emerging again. Joe had an adjustment almost every day he was with us. I am an English major and love poetry; so did Joe, so many days I would quote poetry for him and he really loved that. His favorite, as is mine, is William Wordsworths, The Daffodils. The funny thing was he never made the connection to his adjustments and the recovery of his health. No matter how many times I talked to him to explain that his recovery was from the nervous system healing as a result of the adjustments, it never registered for him. It was as if he had an invisible bubble around his mind that dissolved anything about Chiropractic. The thing he talked about and so appreciated about me was the poetry. As he got stronger and better I continued his daily adjustments and by the end of the year he was well enough to go out and get a job waiting tables. Joe was also a beautiful singer with a talent that would rival Broadway. He felt that if he had a chance to have his dream he would have to go to New York. The year was such a delightful recovery he decided to make the move. He was strong and vital. He looked great and felt great, a true testament to Chiropractic.

As Joe was leaving for New York it was bittersweet for me. There he stood before me radiant and proud, I took his face in my hands, looked deeply in his eyes and asked him, "Joe promise me one thing". "Sure Carol, anything." "Promise me you will find a Chiropractor the day you get into New York." Oh, yes he sheepishly answered. I knew then it was over. You know when someone says they will do something, but yet you know it's just empty words. I felt more troubled with that exchange than I had the first day I saw him at Grady. He left for New York and in two months he was dead. I never saw him again. Of course he did not find a Chiropractor. This stupefied disbelief swallowed me up. I couldn't imagine how someone could live through this recovery day in and day out, adjustment after adjustment and not get that the adjustments were healing his body. After the anger and grief settled down for me I was grateful. Grateful for the last wondrous year that he would never have had without the mysterious and powerful expression of Chiropractic and grateful for me for all the blessings I received from being with Joe. To this day whenever I quote The Daffodils, I have a sweet remembrance.

Carol Billingsley, D.C.
Covington GA, USA
healtoday@aol.com

CHAPTER
THREE

Symptom Based Care vs. Cause Based Care

Chapter 3.

Symptom Based Care vs. Cause Based Care

The terms *diagnosis* and *treatment* belong to the traditional medical practice[1] and lead to *symptom-based care*. Today, better knowledge though neuroscience is moving health fields toward *cause-based care*.

The statement of caused-based care begs the question: What is Cause? When we look at traditional approaches in healthcare, we find they are based on signs and symptoms to form a diagnosis. Once a diagnosis (disease name) has been established, then the treatment is applied. This approach is reflected in current medical practice: patient complains (symptoms), and then various tests are done which produce signs that lead to a drug or procedure that are indicated as the treatment for this pattern (disease). We have come to accept this as typical practice, and over time it has become the standard by which all care is measured. The effectiveness of the treatment is based on the reduction of the signs and symptoms. This is the foundation of so called *evidence-based care*[2]. While this is an important concept, what has been missed with evidence-based care is the true need for establishing the cause of the signs and symptoms. Cause-based care would require that there is evidence the cause of the pain is changing. These are critical differences. Drug companies only require limited proof[3,4] (length of time for testing has been cut by 2/3rds) as to the success of their products which are directed toward symptom-based care. If the symptoms are reduced, the treatment is considered successful -Never mind that other symptoms appear as a direct effect of the drug.

---

1   Medicine - The science of diagnosing, treating, or preventing disease and other damage to the body or mind. The American Heritage® Medical Dictionary Copyright © 2007, 2004

2   Evidence-based health care is the conscientious use of current best evidence in making decisions about the care of individual patients or the delivery of health services. Current best evidence is up-to-date information from relevant, valid research about the effects of different forms of health care, the potential for harm from exposure to particular agents, the accuracy of diagnostic tests, and the predictive power of prognostic factors.

3   FDA Medical Officers Report Lower Standards Permit Dangerous Drug Approvals- December 2, 1998 Peter Lurie, M.D., M.P.H.Sidney M. Wolfe, M.D.

4   The Pharmaceutical Industry - Martin Donohoe, MD, FACPPublic Health and Social Justice Website -http://www.phsj.org - martindonohoe@phsj.org

What modern medicine now has is symptom-based care, not cause-based. As research continues to produce a greater understanding of the role of the stress response as it relates to the cause of disease, health professionals around the world are being forced to revisit their approaches to patient care.

The great challenge in moving the public to a better understanding of health care vs. illness care lies in the depth of two factors.

1. The power of the medical/pharmacology juggernaut and its control over public education. This dates back to the late 1800s when the golden age of science, backed by the science industry, actually had the government pass a ruling that the education system was to be based on the philosophy of reductionism[5]. As the medical /pharmacology industry is totally founded on this theory, the control of the future course of education and health care in North America was set.

2. The public education system had to then follow the above ruling so that public action regarding healthcare would follow what we have been taught. This shift was guaranteed by a wealthy lobby[6] that offered funds to universities to teach the new science. The universities that stayed with old traditions failed to continue op-

---

5   1862 - The First Morrill Act, also known as the "Land Grant Act" becomes law. It donates public lands to states, the sale of which will be used for the "endowment, support, and maintenance of at least one college where the leading object shall be, without excluding other scientific and classical studies and including military tactics, to teach such branches of learning as are related to agriculture and the mechanic arts, in order to promote the liberal and practical education of the industrial classes in the several pursuits and professions in life." Many prominent state universities can trace their roots to this forward-thinking legislation.

An attempt or tendency to explain a complex set of facts, entities, phenomena, or structures by another, simpler set: "For the last 400 years science has advanced by reductionism ... The idea is that you could understand the world, all of nature, by examining smaller and smaller pieces of it. When assembled, the small pieces would explain the whole"(John Holland).

American educational policy and reductionist science: The basis for educational policy in the American educational system is the paradigm of reductionist science or 'reductionism' .basic assumptions. Consistent with reductionist science, 'scientific' observation and inquiry excludes the observer's subjective participation. The scientific perception of 'reality' has been conceived in the context of the objective detachment of the observer. Consistent with the belief in the necessary detachment of the observer, the individual's 'inner reality' has been invalidated as a source of knowledge.

The Shifting Worldview: Toward a More Holistic Science"Reductionistic science, superb for the prediction-and-control task for which it was designed, has mistakenly been elevated by modern society to the position of a worldview. The time seems right for insistence on a holistic science, based on new metaphysical foundations, within which present positivistic, reductionistic science is a limiting case."(Willis Harman.. Holistic Education Review. vol.5 no.3 1992. pp 59-64)

6   1867 - After hearing of the desperate situation facing schools in the south, George Peabody funds the two-million-dollar Peabody Education Fund to aid public education in southern states.

erating. The new order was now in control of information and education. The education now established that the medical / pharmacology model was the only model in health issues and other choices were basically eliminated. Any outside challenge to this model continues to be met with disregard and scorn. Even when proof is presented in which some aspect of current medical concepts are shown to be incorrect or dangerous, the level of indoctrination creates a wall of resistance that can include unethical actions of misinformation and direct attacks to discredit the new information.

3. The Wilk's[7] case is a primary example of how far the medical/pharmacology industry is willing to go to protect their control over the public's right to know. The American Medical Association was directly involved in providing misinformation, slander and restrictive trade action against the chiropractic profession and was found guilty of these actions in the 1970s.

However, even with this court ruling against them, little has changed. Knocking a giant off its pedestal is not an easy task. Currently the medical profession is using scare tactics regarding the so-called danger of cervical adjustments causing strokes in spite of all the research that shows the contrary position[8]. When one looks at the statistics on preventable deaths due to medical malpractice, one has to question the motives and ethics of this misinformation. In case you are not aware of the medical malpractice statistics, the following information is from the "Institute of Medicine" issued on March 1, 2001 in a report titled "Crossing the Quality Chasm: A New Health System for the 21st Century". The IOM is a non-profit advisory organization and is the same agency that reported in 1999 that medical errors (wrong diagnosis, wrong treatment) were killing 98,000 people every year.

So let's get this straight:

- Medical malpractice is the third leading cause of death in the

---

7   Chiropractors sue AMA for antitrust - Wilks v. American Medical Association, 895 F.2d 352 (7th Cir. 1990) UNITED STATES COURT OF APPEALS FOR THE SEVENTH CIRCUIT Nos. 87-2672, 87-2777 - 1990.C07.41521 <http://www.versuslaw.com>; 895 F.2d 352 decided: February 7, 1990

8   Chiropractors don't raise stroke risk, study saysCaroline Alphonso- From Saturday's Globe and Mail - January 19, 2008 at 12:53 AM EST

United States.

- Medical malpractice kills more people than handguns and car accidents

- We spend over a trillion dollars a year on this "health care"

- We spend $75 billion a year on drugs (Legal drugs)

- We spend another $76 billion a year cleaning up the problems those drugs cause (Legal drugs)

- While these are 2001 statistics, they have not improved; in fact, they have gotten worse.

Further, The Journal of the American Medical Association published information regarding medical doctor caused death which stated that "180,000 die each year partly as a result of iatrogenic injury, the equivalent of 3 jumbo-jet crashes every 2 days."[9]

Can you imagine what would happen if an airline had this level of deaths due to crash statistics?

It is the hard facts that show medically modeled symptom-based care has not worked! It is past time for a new approach in healthcare

---

9   Iatrogenic injury -JAMA- Dec.21,1994, Vol.272, #.23, P1851

Chapter 3 - Things to Consider

☞ Do you have a better understanding of the foundation of disease?

☞ Which approach do you think/feel, is a better way to health? 1. Wait for asymptom to develop to provide a foundation for a diagnosis or 2. Test to see if the systems are working correctly before the symptoms occur.

☞ Are you aware that your entire education has been based on reductionism and how this has influenced your health decisions?

☞ Have you ever heard of the "Wilk's" case?

☞ Do you think that modern medicine has all the answers and is the only authority in the health field?

☞ Were you aware of the organized medical action to eradicate chiropractic?

☞ Were you aware of the research that shows the minimal risk of chiropractic adjustment of the cervical spine?

☞ Did you know about the numbers of deaths directly attributed to medical malpractice?

The Fire Fighter's Heart

Dave was a 63 year old gentleman. He had been a fire-fighter and now worked designing new fire engines. He had been a long term patient who came about every 4 weeks - whenever his neck got stiff. We'd talked about more wellness-focused care & maybe seeing him more frequently, but this hadn't been a priority for Dave - only the stiff neck. His son's partner was expecting his first grandchild soon.

In 2010 he decided to have a big health kick and lost 50-odd kilos. In December 2010, he missed his appointment and his wife called to say he was in hospital. He'd been having multiple silent Myocardial Infarctions (Heart attacks) and was now in heart failure.

You need to have 17% heart function remaining to be eligible to have a pacemaker put in. Dave's heart measured at only 11%. So, he was sent home in March with less than 11% heart function to put his affairs in order.

He emailed me –because he was too weak to talk - about whether these wellness ideas we'd discussed might help him. I said that I didn't really know, but if his brain & body were working better, he'd heal if he was able and he had nothing to lose. We use the Neuroinfiniti assessment tool from Neurologically Based Chiropractic, to assess the effects of subluxations on the brain's coordination & control of body functions & over-all health. We assessed Dave's brain wave patterns, the pattern of his heart rate and whether his hand temperature changed predictably. We know all these factors are affected by subluxations of the nervous system.
Based upon Dave's results we developed a plan based around these results that used chiropractic care and targeted nutritional support to address these abnormal results.

His heart function gradually began improving and by August had increased enough to allow surgery for a pacemaker. He had the pacemaker put in in August when he was at 18% heart function (1% over the cut off).

Dave's most recent assessment has his heart function at 22%. The pacemaker has not kicked in to help him once and he's back at work, taking overseas holidays, enjoying being a Grand-dad etc. He has a whole new lease on life. His cardiologist has never seen this happen from 11% before.

Chiropractic care really did save Dave's life and I feel so honoured that I got to be part of that experience for him & his family. This is one of those miracles that is based in science, but still feels miraculous!"

Louise Hockley BSc.(Syd), MChiroprac(Macq)
Chiropractor Level 1, 50 The Terrace, Wellington, New Zealand
www.chiro.co.nz

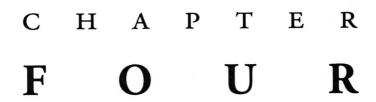

C H A P T E R
F O U R

Misdirected Medical Health Concepts

Chapter 4.

Misdirected Medical Health Concepts

The information in Chapter Two establishes the fact that the current medical model isn't working the way we had hoped. The statistics continue to show that the system is flawed and that there must be some better way to obtain a healthy lifestyle. As presented to this point, the problem is a double-edged sword. One edge is that in order to change the direction of our health attitudes, we first must address the education system which locks us into a reductionism mind set. This mind set is reinforced by "Big Pharma" through their billion dollar advertising campaigns. The second edge is the need to present an option to the current system. Here is the challenge: money not only speaks, it controls our society. Any attempt to present an option to the medical system and the drug cartel is met with Machiavellian tactics.

Well supported information on alternative approaches[1] to a non-medical model lifestyle is available and many people have already opted out of the drug-based symptom care program. You will simply not see these options advertised on TV or see ads for them in magazines

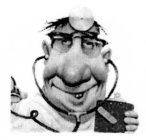

I was watching TV one night. There was a medical doctor speaking about a book called "The End of Illness" he had just published. I got very interested in what he was going to say. He seemed as if he was a bright guy and was talking about how we've been doing health care all wrong. He said we have been treating the symptoms and not looking at the whole body and how it responds. He said, "We know that the biggest culprit in all illness is inflammation." Inflammation is the first level of response to an injury. What he was saying was that inflammation was the big culprit – the cause of illness! He was so excited about this information; however, his solution to the

1   A New Breed Of Healers - John Greenwald Time, April 16, 2001

problem was that everybody should be taking an aspirin a day. Aspirin is an anti-inflammatory, so with his solution in mind, it must mean the body just doesn't produce enough aspirin. Here we have a medical doctor on a main TV channel voicing his great knowledge, stating that the solution to illness is more aspirin. I did not note to see if Bayer was a sponsor of the broadcast. This is nothing short of potion peddling, and it is not an isolated incident!

For decades, billions of research dollars have been poured into the study of bacteria and viruses as the cause of ill health and disease. The results have produced more medicines and treatments, but with failing results! We now have more listed diseases and so many drugs that no one can keep track. The average today is for everyone over 50 to be on 4 to 5 different drugs with the general concept being that this is normal. IT ISN'T! I've actually been confronted by medical personnel telling me that there must be something wrong with me because at age 71, I'm not on any meds. What is going on? There has to be a better way. Iatrogenic disease (doctor caused) has grown at an exponential rate. While we are living longer, the quality of life has diminished. We are now offering drugs to counteract the drugs we are already taking, which is a reason for a 70 year old to be on 4 to 7 different drugs[2]. Medical specialists are only focused on their own areas and communication between them is poor at best. The medical system is financially breaking the country, let alone individuals without expensive medical insurance. A book published in Canada called "Squandering Billions"[3] effectively describes the incredible mismanagement of today's medical healthcare business.

2   Drugs and the Elderly: Practical Considerations - C. Bree Johnston MD MPH   SF VAMC/UCSF -UCSF Division of
     Geriatrics Primary Care Lecture Series May 2001

3   "Squandering Billions"– Gary Bannerman, Don Nixdorf, D.C. ISBN 0-88839-602-X – Hancock Publishers LTD.

Doug's story

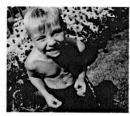

"Doug" was a normal healthy boy until he had his vaccination shots. Within 24 hours he went into anaphylactic shock[4] which resulted in severe nervous system damage. When I first saw Doug he could not walk well, and if he tried to run he would fall. He was extremely hyperactive, could not speak beyond one or two words, and was more than the family could handle. The parents were exhausted. The medical answer was to first off deny it had anything to do with the vaccines; and second, was to place him on meds that were damaging his liver. He was on a downhill spiral. I started him on chiropractic care and after a few months he was a different child. He could talk and run. He was off all but one of the medical drugs and had returned to being a wonderful young normal boy. During the time of his chiropractic care, the family's MD and the school were pressuring the parents to have Doug's younger sister vaccinated, knowing full well the family history. These are the people in control of the information and guidelines of healthcare in the world today. Where is common sense; and an even more powerful question, where are their morals?

The end of the story however takes a nasty turn. I left practice in 1995 and with that Doug's parents stopped the chiropractic care. About two years later, I received notice that Doug had died. To this day, I have a challenge with what happened to that wonderful life. First off, the so-called health system doesn't consider the adverse effects of vaccinations and just views Doug as a low incident of negative response. It is all well and good to think of this type of reaction as "a few" until it is a child you know. Everyday children are challenged with this type of medical intervention but the statistics are never shown to the public. If you would like more information, there is a book called "A Shot in the Dark" by Harris H. Coulter and Barbara Loe Fisher. Just read the

---

4   Risk of anaphylaxis after vaccination of children and adolescents. Bohlke K, Davis RL, Marcy SM, Braun MM, DeStefano F, Black SB, Mullooly JP, Thompson RS; Vaccine Safety Datalink Team. - Pediatrics. 2003 Oct;112(4):815-20. - Center for Health Studies, Group Health Cooperative, Seattle, Washington 98101-1448, USA.

reviews and you will see why this is such an important issue.

Today everyone seems to view vaccination as a standard, safe, procedure. What you don't know is:

- What is actually in the vaccine[5] that you inject directly into your system, bypassing the first levels of defenses of your immune system.

- The statistics used by science that call the severe damage, such as Doug's, as incidental. The numbers are far greater than the public knows and for Doug's parents, far from incidental.

This level of hidden damage isn't just about childhood vaccines - it includes all forms, from shingles to the yearly flu shots. Lives are involved so be sure to gather all the information you can before just following the ads you hear on television. This is really a case of "buyer beware!" Remember that there is no such thing as a free flu shot - Big Pharma gets paid![6]

Chapter 4 - Things to Consider

Are you aware:

☞ Of limited thinking within the medical community? (Such as: if inflammation is the problem, the body must be short of aspirin!)

☞ That taking medicine is just to be expected?

☞ The majority of meds are taken because of the direct effect of some previous med?

---

5   Vaccine ingredients a. Micro-organisms, either bacteria or viruses, thought to be causing certain infectious diseases and which the vaccine is supposed to prevent. These are whole-cell proteins or just the broken-cell protein envelopes, and are called antigens.
b. Chemical substances which are supposed to enhance the immune response to the vaccine, called adjuvants. c. Chemical substances which act as preservatives and tissue fixatives, which are supposed to halt any further chemical reactions and putrefaction (decomposition or multiplication) of the live or attenuated (or killed) biological constituents of the vaccine."--VieraScheibner

6   Pharmacies Profit from Dangerous Flu Shot, Disrupt Medical Records - Lisa Garber - Infowars.com September 24, 2012

☞ There is solid proof that questions the value of vaccinations; and that children have died or been brain damaged because of vaccination?

☞ Who is responsible for these damaged children?

☞ Who makes money from the vaccination program in schools?

☞ If your child is vaccinated and, therefore, is supposedly immune, why worry about some other child not vaccinated being a threat to you?

Failure-to-Thrive Infant - Mary Ann

One day when I was in my son's school, the administrator came up to me with her grandson in her arms. She told me how he was on the way to the hospital but she had begged her daughter to give the boy to her for the day. She had felt that there was going to be some way that she was going to get him help. For the most part, he had stopped eating. He was able to get down three ounces of formula a day for the past few days. He was three ounces under his birth weight and he was five weeks old. He was a failure-to-thrive infant and she was obviously scared. She had followed her heart and against all the pressure to get him into a neonatal unit, she was standing in front of me asking for help.

She had known of some of the work I had done with infants, handed the baby to me and asked me if I would help. I nodded an enthusiastic yes and set about examining him. He was extremely lethargic, not moving and seemed in a semi-consciousness state. I did my exam on him and found that he couldn't bend like he should be able to and that when I put my finger in his mouth his tongue was stuck in the back of his throat, poking my finger like a wood pecker, tapping a tree. The roof of his mouth, the palate, was also disfigured. One side had slightly dropped down, creating a rift between the right and left sides of the roof of the mouth.

From this I knew, when he tried to drink he wasn't able to get his tongue involved and then not able to suck on the nipple of the bottle. He would also have had a sour stomach, because the gag reflex had moved from the back of his throat to the top of his palate. So every time the nipple was rubbing the palate he was gagging, causing an upset stomach. When I told her all of this her mouth dropped open with wonderment. No one had been able to examine him and then tell her what was happening to him. The medical world was at a loss and so was the family. Relief spread across her face as she started to anticipate that I may help this little fellow. A smile crossed my face as I let her know that I would start working on him immediately.

For the next hour I worked on his body and brought him back to balance, via gentle chiropractic infant adjustments, infant myofascial unwinding along with cranial work. The grandmother was crying as I was working on him because she could see how loving the work was and that her grandson was responding positively. After the hour was over, I retested him and sure enough his tongue was extending and he was able to use it again. The gag reflex had gone to the back of his throat and his range of motion had gone to normal. The only problem was with the tongue. It was coming out to the front of his mouth, but it still was not curling around my finger. It basically stayed flat. This is important because he needed the curling ability so that he could get a good suction on the nipple. Many mothers are frustrated because their baby doesn't latch on to her nipple and are not able to nurse. A simple chiropractic adjustment would heal the baby and all frustration would be gone.

I told the grandmother that he was better, bring him home and let him eat, be with his mother and watch. I told her not to wait to bring him to the hospital if he didn't start to eat right away. If he was better, I would want to see him again the next day for a tune up. She was happy as she bundled him up to bring him home. I received a phone call three hours later with yelps of joy in the background that the baby had just eaten four ounces of food without throwing up. I smiled. Four hours later another phone call, this time in tears when she relayed to me that the baby had just eaten seven ounces of formula and his eyes were open and responding to his mother. My heart leapt with joy as I took a deep breath and thanked God for what I and lots of other chiropractors know, healing comes from within and if the brain is reconnected to the body, health is possible and probable. My only sorrow was the thousands of other infants that needed similar help.

The next day the grandparent brought him to me and he looked like a different baby. His eyes were open and his arms were active. He looked at me and I felt a wave of gratitude flow from him to me. I gave him a kiss on his check and said, "You are welcome my sweet little one." I checked his tongue and it still wasn't able to curl. I worked on him some more and sure enough by the end of the session his tongue was able to create a strong suction and function just like it was meant to. The gag reflex was still in the back of his throat. I sent him off in perfect health. The grandmother kept me informed of his progress and he quickly gained the weight and thrived.

Mary Ann Luckett, D.C.
Covington GA, USA
healtoday@aol.com

CHAPTER
FIVE

**The Historical Events that Shaped
the Chiropractic Profession**

Chapter 5.

The Historical Events that Shaped
the Chiropractic Profession

The first unfortunate development of chiropractic lies in the timing of its founding in 1895. During this time, the so-called scientific world took a turn in a totally opposite direction from the foundations of chiropractic. The primary philosophical position in the previous scientific world had been vitalistic in nature (that there was a vital force in life beyond the chemical and physical); but during the late 1800s a new scientific belief, or philosophy, called "atomism" or "reductionism" (life was only chemical or physical and by understanding the parts, we could then control life) became the center of attention. Chiropractic was, and still is, one-hundred percent a vitalistic-based profession. It was unfortunate timing, as the scientific world of that time totally rejected any possibility or potential for chiropractic, and medicine turned to the reductionistic belief that gave them control as discussed in Chapter 2.

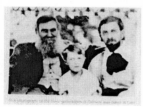

D.D. Palmer David Palmer , B.J, Palmer

The vast majority of people have no idea why the two professions oppose one another, nor do they have any idea of the concepts of the two different philosophies. The great challenge here is that people make their health choices on one of these two approaches without any real knowledge of the philosophical foundations of their decision.

The limited understanding of neurological function at the time of D.D. Palmer's founding theories of chiropractic (1895) gave rise to the conclusion that moving a vertebra in the spine altered body function, and this was the basis for "vertebral subluxation (VS) as the cause of disease"[1] for chiropractic. While D.D. later moved to a more complete

---

1   "Reflex effects of vertebral subluxations: the peripheral nervous system. An update.".Bolton P (2000). J

understanding of the neurological role, the "VS" definition remained the unique selling point for the chiropractic practitioner.

The founding family of the chiropractic profession had its own internal struggles with a father/son battle that had a great effect on the direction of chiropractic in the early years. D.D felt pushed aside with his son's ability to market chiropractic from a somewhat different point of view. The battle was significant enough to create a split within the profession as to the scope of practice included in chiropractic practice. Even today there is a difference from state to state and country to country as to what chiropractors can do and what chiropractic care includes in their offices.[2]

These internal challenges, along with the challenges from medicine, have not helped in either public opinion or the organization of the profession. The public's exposure to the profession has been left to knowledge through experience, or word of mouth. Due to the variety of approaches within the profession, the experience in one chiropractic office could be totally different from another. The one area that was similar, however, was the focus on the importance of the spinal bones (vertebra). It was the central body part in the explanation of chiropractic to both the mechanical and the philosophical positioned doctors of chiropractic. The problem with the use of dry specimen spines in explaining chiropractic was that we became known as bone doctors or worse, back-crackers. The importance of the relationship between the chiropractic adjustment and the nervous system was replaced with the importance of moving bones and joints.

The science of the 1890's and early 1900's was not developed enough to offer support to the chiropractic theory. Under the leadership of B.J. Palmer, considered to be the developer of chiropractic, the profession rallied around a philosophy of chiropractic. The philosophy of chiropractic was developed to protect the profession from attacks by

---

Manipulative PhysiolTher 23 (2): 101-3. PMID 10714535 Professor Philip S. Bolton, School of Biomedical Sciences at University of Newcastle, Australia writes in JMPT, "The traditional chiropractic vertebral subluxation hypothesis proposes that vertebral misalignment causes illness, disease, or both. This hypothesis remains controversial."

2   Chiropractic in the United States:Training, Practice, and Research   Chapter V: Licensure and Legal Scope of Practice – Ruth Sandefur, DC, PhD; Ian D. Coulter, PhDwww.chirobase.org/05RB/AHCPR/05.html

the medical profession, and established chiropractic as separate from medicine. This philosophy was the moving force of the profession until the early 1960s and lead to a devoted band of chiropractic followers. There are many books on the philosophy of chiropractic, but because of the lack of any scientific proof, outside of great results, the profession looked more like a cult than a true healing art. Any results were dismissed as anecdotal and the profession ridiculed. Even though publicly challenged, the remarkable results from chiropractic care continued the profession's existence. The level of knowledge and education of practitioners increased and from this developed both the art (application of chiropractic techniques), and a chiropractic lifestyle.

The profession, still lacking the vital link between the adjustment and the results, started to look at explanations that could be supported with current science. This created a shift away from the neurological construct developed by D.D. and B.J. Palmer to a more mechanical model involving posture, the spine and joint mechanics. Even though the nervous system was at the center of the chiropractic intent, the focus on the joints of the spine set the direction of the profession until 2005 when the first paper was published providing evidence of the chiropractic adjustment's direct effect on brain function.

Today, the shift to the mechanical model has again created a split in the profession with some chiropractors following the mechanical model (which is a shift to the medical model) focused on the spine and movement, while others remain dedicated to the philosophical model (the Vitalistic model)

A new model has emerged which brings the two together. Today, we are beginning to understand how and why the adjustment has achieved such remarkable results over the years. The development of the computer has played a big role in the emergence of scientific support for chiropractic. The advent of the Electroencephalograph (EEG) and recent studies have provided evidence of the connection between the chiropractic adjustment and alterations in central nervous system function. The new model is called Neurologically Based Chiropractic. (NBC).

Chapter 5 - Things to Consider

☞ Do you understand why your chiropractic experience can differ from chiropractor to chiropractor?

☞ Can you see how medicine and chiropractic differ in their approaches to health?

☞ Do you see why medicine and chiropractic are at odds?

☞ Do you understand how chiropractors became known as back doctors?

☞ Can you see that there is more to the chiropractic approach than has been told in the past?

Lost Boys

He walked in without a smile, staying very close to his mom as if he did not want anyone to notice him. He didn't speak much nor could he balance well, ride a bike, or engage with other six year-old boys. So many boys seem to have lost their wild-at-heart spirit and here was one more who just joined the team. He was not able to follow much of the physical exam and the neurological component intensified his withdrawn state. My journey with children has illustrated a reflection of research I read years ago: "over the age of thirty increased risk of adult-onset disease, but under thirty they are simply not wiring up as expected", (Hansen and Butrum, 1976). Early in practice, as I am sure most of you have seen too, many adults are not well. And now, everyone knows of a child who is altered in their development or has been labeled Autistic, AD(H)D, OCD, ODD.......LMNOP. The label helps some navigate their child through school or medical services. Regardless of the label, what is happening to generations of children is a travesty.

This lost boy began his time here on earth under the neglectful watch of his biological mother. He was taken from her because he had pneumonia, then placed in an orphanage where she had one year to return to pick him up. She never came back. He placed for adoption and was received by two incredible parents. His journey has been difficult, trying, restraining, removed, nothing short of stressful. However, now after 1.5 years, he tells us about his train room, he can read labels and knows what foods support him and which ones he needs to stay away from, rides a bike, and just began playing football. We still have work ahead with his social skills which are still under-developed but wow, what a different little boy stands in front of us today.

My practice follows the progressive development for the pediatric neurological system; included in this process are reflexes. Reflexes are the primitive foundation and rudimentary training for all neurological development. The nervous system should integrate this training and then inhibit the reflex. Inhibition does not mean the reflexes are gone but rather a foundation for the next level of maturation to bloom. If a reflex does not inhibit, the next step in progression is altered. The severity of the alteration is unique and individual to the person.

Each person, child or adult, may demonstrate altered behavior or skill. The difference between children and adults are their prior experiences influencing the maturation of physiological function or behavior. Children have a limited base of interpretation, while an adult, speculating that the adult did move through progressive development as expected, now has many many files of data in their brain to pull from for function and behavior. However, if the insult to the adult is great enough, stroke, heart attack, emotional breakdown, the adult too can return to primal function for re-education. Most therapeutic modalities focus to re-educate through repetitive motor planning to regain close to normal function. Unfortunately, children under developed cannot pull from something that does not exist. Working with the lost boys has reminded me how a veterinarian must feel like. The animals come in and the doctor relies heavily on what the owner conveys. I must listen to the parents, and in fact the *history is my greatest tool in building the blue print of each and every child. The history of this little boy painted a picture of initially not being wanted, discarded, and without a concern.*

The earliest component of development includes a set of reflexes known as the withdrawal reflexes. These reflexes prime the nervous system for survival. As the withdrawal reflexes mature, they will actually be known as the crossed-extensor reflex for pain. The possibility of "getting stuck" in a reflex, changing one's compass of developmental direction is most intriguing to me. Did he get stuck? Where was this underlying directional pull taking him inside of his little body and his relationship with the rest of the world? How could I objectively evaluate and monitor changes that his parents would accept and follow?

An amazing instrument exists in the chiropractic profession known as the NeuroInfiniti, and its developer and leader Dr. Richard Barwell are truly a blessing to our profession. The NeuroInfiniti measures the stress response inside an individual. Now before launching into the data, allow me to connect the stress-response from a reflexive developmental perspective. The second set of reflexes is called the primitive reflexes. The first primitive reflex is known as the Moro reflex which will later develop into the adult startle response.

The Moro reflex comes on the ninth week of gestation priming arousal for the sleep-wake cycle, CO_2/O_2 balance, and the sympathetic nervous system. The Moro reflex should inhibit at four-month post-natal development. If this reflex remains facilitated the child presents with altered sleep patterns, too much or too little, altered respiration patterns, too much or too little, and altered sympathetic engagement, too much or too little. These altered patterns are exactly what I can see from the NeuroInfiniti Stress Evaluation. In addition, I can tell if the patterns are chronic. Chronic sympathetic stress patterns change bioenergetic pathways during open windows of development.

This little lost boy, during a critical time of data entry, was on his own to interpret the world around him. The physiological and emotional stress changed function. We could measure the component of physiological stress and what was now happening to his system and explain his responses. The NeuroInfiniti demonstrates brain waves and their affect on heart-rate variability, heart rate, respiration, skin conduction, temperature, and muscle tonal responses in the trapezium muscle response to stress. The parents found the information incredibly interesting and practical. Together we changed this child's diet, corrected his physical challenges, and continue to integrate his system with the world around him. The follow-up assessments have identified specific areas still needing additional attention. The information provided by the NeuroInfiniti has improved my abilities as a doctor.

Laura Hanson, D.C., D.I.C.C.P., NDT
Alpharetta GA, USA
originaldevelopment@gmail.com

CHAPTER
SIX

**Is the Body a Self-Correcting,
Self-Healing Entity?**

Chapter 6.
Is the body a self-correcting, self-healing entity?

So now that the rug has been pulled out from under the "germ theory" and the vertebral subluxation as the cause of disease, where does this leave us in the healthcare field? Add to this the effects of prescription drugs and we can see why many are questioning the direction of healthcare. On the one hand we have a system built on self-perpetuating sickness management, and on the other a health art lacking scientific validation. That is until now!

The questions are, "How did we manage to survive before we had modern medicine?" Does the body have the ability and intelligence to know how to survive?

The body has a built in self-correcting system, and while this is true, that it is self-healing, it is true only to a point. There have been many theories in the past including the idea that all we have to do is trust the body and it will always do the right thing. However, once the system has been damaged, the ability to return to ideal is compromised.

When we look at the nervous system, we see there are states of the neurological status quo. A beautifully balanced nervous system can adapt and respond to its environment correctly. An example would be when a bear comes out of the woods and attacks you, you go into the full flight mode, and you run away. When you get away everything returns to normal. That's the ideal stress response situation. If this stress response system starts to break down, there are six different directions that can develop. These six response patterns are less than ideal and will be discussed in later chapters.

When a nervous system becomes overloaded or stressed, there is so much input going on that the system begins to "short circuit." The brain's processing resources become overwhelmed so that these "short circuits" create inappropriate responses.[1] The inappropriate response

---

1   Brain Economics: - Housekeeping Routines in the Brain - Proefschriftterverkrijging van het doctoraat in de

disruptions feed back into the other body systems, which in turn create additional stress on the already overloaded central nervous system.

As the various systems within the body all rely on each other to stay in balance (this is called a closed loop system) these inappropriate response disruptions create an unbalancing of other body functions. The only way the nervous system can warn the individual of the unbalancing is to create signs and/or symptoms. What we now know is that there is a direct relationship between the state of your central nervous system and the signs and symptoms produced.[2] The significance of this knowledge is that we now understand there is a direct link between the stressors in your life, your neurological response, your recovery ability and your illnesses. This is known as the *stress response* and is the emerging field in health science.[3]

All you have to do is go online and do a search for "stress and disease" and you will see that this field is ever expanding. The new understanding of the relationship between stress and disease is changing every form of healthcare.

What we need now is a method of stress response measurement. With objective measurements of the neurophysiological response and recovery during and after a stressful experience, we will have a great deal of valuable information regarding the state of a patient's health. The challenge therein is that we are dealing with a dynamic being, always sensing and adapting. This means that any type of static examination such as x-ray, static para-spinal scanning including EMG thermal and postural scans, or even blood testing only presents information on that patient as a moment in time.

MedischeWetenschappenaan de Rijksuniversiteit Groningen op gezag van de Rector Magnificus, dr. F. Zwarts, in het openbaarteverdedigen op maandag 5 oktober 2009 om 14.45 uur door Paolo Toffaningeboren op 12 maart 1979 teSandrigo, Itali''ePromotores : Prof. dr. A. Johnson Prof. dr. R. de Jong Prof. dr. G.J. ter Horst Copromotor : Dr. S. Martens Beoordelingscommissie : Prof. dr. M. Eimer Prof. dr. B. Hommel Prof. dr. N.M. Maurits ISBN (boek): 978-90-367-3979-5 ISBN (digitaal): 978-90-367-3978-8

2 Health Psychology Meets The Central Nervous System -Dr. Cheryl MacDonald, RN., Psy'D. Health Psychology of San Diego October 5, 2011 in Neur

3 The epidemiology, pathophysiology, and management of psychosocial risk factors in cardiac practiceThe emerging field of behavioral cardiology -American College of Cardiology Foundation Volume 45, Issue 5, March 2005>State-of-the-art paper March 2005

A good example of the challenges of static type tests lies in the typical blood pressure testing. When the testing is done in the doctor's office the "White Coat Syndrome"[4] plays a role in elevating blood pressure. When BP is taken several times outside the doctor's office, a drop in pressure is recorded.

Our lives are complicated and multi-faceted, as are our body's systems and responses. Today any testing must be done over time and under different situations (when possible) to obtain an accurate picture of our body's ability to respond, recover and adapt to stress.

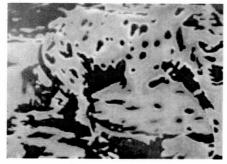

It is rather like looking at a small part of a Salvador Dali painting and thinking that you have seen the entire picture. Note the small picture of the dog. Now see if you can find it in the large painting titled the "Hallucinogenic Toreador".(If you have never experienced Salvador Dali's work, you owe yourself the experience -The Dalí Museum – 1 Dali Street Blvd., St. Petersburg, FL 33701) 727 823 3767

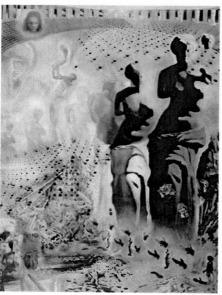

---

4   My Blood Pressure Is Only High at the Doctor's Office: Do I Need Treatment? Craig Weber, M.D., former About.com Guide Updated February 02, 2007

Chapter 6 - Things to Consider

☞ How stressors in life directly affect the balance of the body's systems function.

☞ Stress responses and recovery are the key to understanding our health issues.

☞ Dynamic testing (testing over time and different events) reveals a much better picture of your body's ability to adapt and respond than does a static test (a moment in time) such as an x-ray.

☞ The bigger picture is critical in laying out a course of care.

☞ Salvador Dali was a very strange but incredible artist.

My storey is a long one, but I will try write briefly with the hopes you can interpret and change accordingly for better reading should you wish to use it J should you need more detail or info please let me know.

Firstly I decided to start studying chiropractic after being in my second year of doing a BSc in zoology and having very bad lower back pain that did not resolve with physiotherapy. A family friend suggested chiropractic and after going to the chiropractor I just knew this was what I wanted to do. I soon changed courses.

In my first year of practice, my mom had a nervous breakdown. Her husband was murdered a few years back and her health slowly started deteriorating. She was not treated for this but was only put onto benzodiazepines and provided sleeping tablets. She kept returning to the GP complaining of anxiety and trouble sleeping and he simply upped her dosages. As her health deteriorated she was then placed on meds for her thyroid. She met another man and they moved in together, but this relationship was not a very loving one from his side. His 2 sons lived with them and they treated my mom badly as well. She started self-medicating and eventually turned to alcohol. I had taken her to numerous doctors and psychologists and psychiatrists and eventually she reached a breaking point and had to be admitted.

She was taken off the benzodiazepines cold turkey. She went through a very bad withdrawal where she became psychotic after this incidence and sustained a minor stroke with a very high blood pressure. The medical insurance ran out and she was sent home, where she tried to commit suicide. She was then admitted into a government psychiatric ward and spent a few months there. After many different drug therapies and eventually trying shock therapy, which did not help much for the major depressive disorder but seemed to improve the psychosis, she was released as an outpatient, which meant she stayed at home, but came in every month to be checked and get a new script of medications. This went on for about 2 years, and after seeing many more psychiatrists, they eventually said there was nothing they could do for her.

During this time, I myself had developed some uncomfortable neurologic symptoms and was later diagnosed with MS. I started seeing a neurologically based chiropractor, Dr Ricardo Jorge, and after seeing the biochart on his wall and the MS in the exhausted nervous system state, it all made sense to me! I started listening to Dr Barwell's webinars and became inspired and excited and understood how the stress had affected my health and that of my moms and how we could reverse it. I started going to Dr Jorge regularly and then after hearing about my mom he suggested I bring her in too. After 3 months of care, my mom started to change. At the start of her care, she was like a zombie, she did not talk much, was not alert, could not hold a conversation and slept and smoked all day long.

She was still staying with the man who she had met a couple years back and his 2 sons and their little toddlers. This was not a good loving environment at all and my mom was emotionally and mentally abused but she would not acknowledge that or accept help from myself. Eventually after about 6 or so months of care, after my mom was physically assaulted by this man's son, she called a friend and told her that she didn't want to stay there anymore. My mom was not able to see this or do this before she started care.

She did not call her friends or see them at all. When asked how things were all she said every time was "fine ". That is when my brother and I stepped in and took her out of that situation. It has been a tough long road to recovery. She has since been diagnoses with diabetes as well but is managing that very well. She still gets adjusted once to twice a week now, and every week I see more change and improvement in my mom. At one stage I felt that I had lost my dad (to death) as well as my mom (although she was alive physically, there was no soul, and she was as good as dead) and all I wished for was to have my mom back! And I can now say that I have my mom back!

She engages in conversation, and actually askes me now what is going on in my life as well as takes pride in her appearance, and gets excited about the prospect of the future with grand kids. On my side as well, with my on-going chiropractic adjustments, my health has been great! I feel that I have overcome this diagnosis of MS and been able to reverse it completely through the teachings and treatments of neurologically based chiropractic, all brought about through seeing Dr Jorge and being introduced to and listen to Dr Barwell. I wish every single person could get under care! This world would be another place!!!

Kind regards
Dr Nicole Puchner
Chiropractor (MTech SA, MCASA)
DOCS@WORK, 99 Michelle Avenue
Randhart, Alberton Tel/fax : 011 869 190

CHAPTER
SEVEN

The Emerging Health Field

Chapter 7.

The Emerging Health Field

Today we have research that connects the nervous system with the immune system, but this is a relatively new discovery. It wasn't until the 1980s that medical research finally found these two systems directly connected[1]. Until then, the medical position was that the nervous and immune systems were totally independent body systems. The importance of this point is that until we understood the relationship between the nervous system and the immune system, there was no foundation to establish *cause* beyond signs and symptoms. This simple point was a major point of contention between the medical and chiropractic professions for almost a hundred years. The chiropractic profession's position was that every system was controlled by the nervous system. Medicine attacked chiropractic as a nonsense uninformed cult and when the neurological and immune system relationship was "discovered" in 1980, there was not one mention from medicine admitting that Chiropractors were right all along.

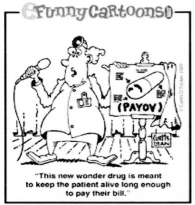

"This new wonder drug is meant to keep the patient alive long enough to pay their bill."

The 1990s were known as the decade of the brain[2]. During these ten years, more knowledge was gathered about the brain and its function than had been known in all the previous years. Now, in this decade, the focus is on "consciousness"[3] and again, the research shows that the role the nervous system plays in our ability to be healthy has changed the concepts of

1   Healing and the Mind by Bill Moyers ... from David Felton, MD, Ph.D from the U of Rochester School of Medicine on "The Brain and the Immune System"

2   Decade of the brain. An agenda for the nineties. M Goldstein - West J Med. 1994 September; 161(3): 239–241. PMCID: PMC1011403

3   in the first decade of the 21st century, the study of consciousness has become a highly dynamic field,- Institute of Neurosciences, Mental Health and Addiction (Canada)

health and disease.

Why don't you know about this? The answer is simple: it doesn't involve the sale of drugs and has created a major dilemma for the medical profession. The medical profession has become so invested in drug based therapy that it is virtually impossible for them to shift to a new understanding. Today the drug companies have bypassed the Medical Doctor and advertise directly to the public. Wall Street has become the new drug pusher[4,5].

While this drug obsession has been developing, there has been a group of researchers working in a different direction. Over the last 50 years there has been a group of PhDs getting fantastic results by working on how people can change their brain function using biofeedback and/or neurofeedback[6]. These researchers have created a way to objectively measure changes in nervous system function and the resulting effect on people's health. The research over the last 20 years on brain activity has revealed that brain function is the controller of your health patterns. When we look at both research groups (the neuroscience and the biofeedback) a completely new understanding of the cause of disease and illness takes shape. New knowledge is not always met with welcoming arms!

"Innovators are seldom received with joy. For every crossroads of the future there are a thousand self-appointed guardians of the past". Dr. Allan Beer M.D. Fertility Expert

In 1977, Dr. John Knowles, President of the Rockefeller Foundation wrote - "80% of serious illnesses seem to develop when the individual feels helpless or hopeless" … "over 99 percent of us are born healthy and made sick as a result of human misbehavior".[7] In 2000 a paper produced by the National Institute of Health (NIH) stated: "But in the last decade, scientists like Dr. Esther Sternberg, director of the

4   Big Pharma Paying Out Huge Settlements In Marketing Cases By Dunstan Prial Published November 23, 2011 FOXBusiness

5   Drug Pushers…They're closer than you think!June 20, 2012 By Dr Sarahvitalmoms.com/drug-pusherstheyre-closer-than-you-think/

6   The Byers Neurotherapy Reference Library – Second Edition – Alvah P. Byers EdD 1995 AAPB ISBN 1-887114-04-1

7   Dr. John Knowles, President of the Rockefeller Foundation wrote in DAEDALUS, (Winter, 1977)

Integrative Neural Immune Program at NIH's National Institute of Mental Health (NIMH), have been rediscovering the links between the brain and the immune system".[8]

It has now become obvious that when it comes to disease, in either prevention of, or creation of, the relationship between the nervous system and the immune system is the key factor, and not viruses and/or bacteria. The billions or trillions spent on disease research, such as cancer, has only produced limited results with the primary benefit being early detection.

The previous chapters have been laying the ground work by providing facts that demonstrate how the concepts that have guided medicine and chiropractic in the past are no longer relevant. Time has provided the opportunity for us to examine the flaws in both of these fields when it comes to considering the long term assessment of theory and conclusion. The old adage of "If it ain't broke, don't fix it" seems to be in play with both fields. That is until someone can show that they are, in fact, "BROKE." Until the public has access to the real data and facts, it will continue to assume that this is the way the health system works, the ad men and system controllers know best, and that is the way it is.

It is time for this new perspective to become the foundation for not only further research, but more importantly, the entire healthcare system.

Chapter 7 - Things to Consider

☞ There is a direct link between the nervous system, the endocrine system and the immune system.

☞ While chiropractors have been talking about this link for 100 years, medicine said they were wrong until they themselves discovered it in 1980.

☞ Since 1990 we have learned more about the brain and nervous system than all the time before this combined.

---

8   Stress and Disease: New Perspectives - By Harrison Wein, Ph.D. The National Institute of Health - Word on Health - October 2000

CHAPTER
EIGHT

The Role of the Nervous System in Health

Chapter 8.

The Role of the Nervous System in Health

An anatomy textbook, by Lockhart, Hamilton and Fyfe, describes the nervous system this way: "Even in the smallest community of men the activities of different individuals must be coordinated by some 'central authority' for the common good – nature has solved the same problem by creating a controlling system."

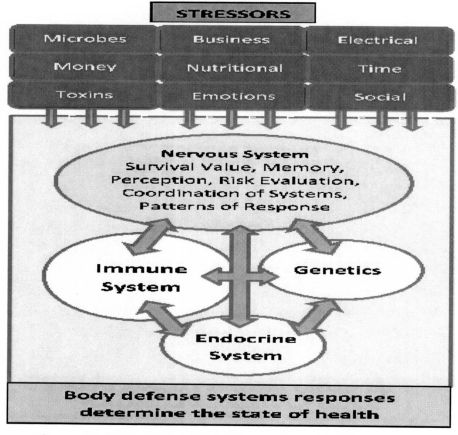

This controlling system (the nervous system) receives information from the environment, both external and internal, sends it to the brain (the central organizing authority) and then the brain sends signals out to the systems of the body to create an appropriate response. We now know that this includes the immune system, whose responsibility it is to protect us from outside influences such as bacteria and viruses. The nervous system has several divisions. It has a sensory division, whose job is to relay information into the brain; and a motor division, which carries action information to the muscles.

There is another nervous system division called the autonomic nervous system, which takes care of the subconscious needs such as heart rate, respiratory rate, temperature, skin moisture, muscle tone, digestion, excretion and many other factors.

About 80 to 90 percent of brain activity is dedicated to just keeping the body running without us ever being aware of the activities. The immune system depends upon the nervous system information to keep us healthy. As the body is considered to be a closed loop system, meaning that all the systems have an influence on one another, it requires a level of balance or harmony to function correctly. Any factor that upsets the controlling system will create disturbances in the other systems, including the immune response, endocrine function (hormones), muscle tone, temperature regulation, respiration rate, heart rate, digestion, reproduction and excretion.

The interaction between the systems must remain within balance, with each part communicating with the other via the nervous system. This balance activity is called *homeostasis*. The concept of homeostasis has been discussed for centuries and has been recognized as a critical component of health.

The current research has altered the concept of homeostasis from a static balance to a dynamic picture of system interaction as the systems respond to every changing environmental influence. The term now being used to express this wonderful life dance is called *allostasis*[1].

The application of reductionism in medicine, treating only one

1   The concept of allostasis in biology and biomedicine. McEwen BS, Wingfield JC. - HormBehav. 2003 Jan;43(1):2-15.Laboratory of Neuroendocrinology, The Rockefeller University, PMID:12614627[PubMed - indexed for MEDLINE]

part, and specific drug usage based on symptoms, has some inherent flaws that explain the ever increasing use of drugs with patients as they age. This increasing drug use is a primary factor in the increasing cost of Medicare and a threat to public health.[2]

Any care program that addresses only one system challenge will un-balance the others. We are seeing this with the addition of prescriptions issued to a patient over time, ending up with the four to seven different drugs by age fifty[3]. These are not short term prescriptions but lifetime programs. Finally the system's balance becomes so disrupted that we see failing health with more expensive care procedures required. The health care in North America is really illness management[4] and there-fore has become the most costly system worldwide. If you are invested in Wall Street drug companies, you will leave your children a good re-turn on your investment, which they will need with the soaring medi-cal costs.

Instead of looking for cheaper drugs, we need to start to deal with the cause of our loss of allostatic balance. Step one is to first under-stand the role of the nervous system in maintaining this balance, and step two is to discover why it has lost control. Step three, and the rea-son for this book, is to learn how to regain control without the damag-ing effects of drugs or surgery.

2   U.S. Health Care Costs = Kaiser Health News Headlines - www.kaiseredu.org/issue-modules/us...costs/background-brief.aspx

3   Prescription Drug Use Continues to Increase: U.S. Prescription Drug Data for 2007-2008 - QiupingGu, M.D., Ph.D.; Charles F. Dillon, M.D., Ph.D.; and Vicki L. Burt, Sc.M., R.N.- - National Center for Health Statistics Brief - Number 42, September 2010

4   ILLNESS BEHAVIOUR - Challenging the Medical Model - Humane Medicine - the Journal of the Art and Sci-ence of Medicine Volume 10 Number 3

Chapter 8 - Things to Consider

☞ Stress directly affects your immune system.

☞ What are the stressors in your life?

☞ The brain (central controlling authority) continually exchanges information with the immune system and the endocrine system.

☞ 80 to 90 percent of brain function is subconscious and is responsible for keeping the systems in balance.

☞ If one part of the closed loop system is challenged, it directly affects other inter-looped systems.

☞ Medical drugs create greater imbalance in the systems.

☞ How many drugs are you currently taking?

☞ Did you find the need to take an additional drug after taking a drug for a previous problem?

☞ America is declining in quality of health.

☞ Big Pharma and the Medical Industrial Complex have built a treatment business for the diseases they create.

CHAPTER

NINE

The Role of the
Immune System

Chapter 9.

The Role of the Immune System

The immune system is our "On Guard 24/7" system. It never sleeps and it will respond to any injury. However, it does not have to wait for injury to happen and will even be kicked into action as a result of a perceived injury or threat. These threats are called stressors and may be as serious as a severe wound, all the way down to a merely perceived (may not be real) threat. The nervous system creates special hormones such as adrenalin and cortisol to stimulate the immune and other systems into action.

The first level of response to a stress (perceived or real) lies within the nervous system, and the immune response is the first to answer the call. There are several levels of activity initiated including: increases in heart rate, respiration rate, blood pressure, sweat gland activity, muscle tone, and platelet production; decreased hand and feet temperatures; and changes in brain wave activity.

In fact, there are many other factors involved, including the release of hormones such as glucagon (pancreas stimulating), glucocorticoids (steroids -metabolism and immune function), and prolactin (pituitary -reproduction suppression). The latest research and books being published on the effects of "stressors" and "stress-response" clearly explain the connection between neurological function, immune system involvement and health patterns.

I recommend *Why Zebras Don't Get Ulcers: an updated guide to stress, stress-related diseases and coping*, by Robert M. Sapolsky[1]. It's an excellent piece of work. He picks up where Hans Selye left off back in the 60s with his book on STRESS. I recall reading Selye's book in college and I thought he had the answer. He finally started to understand why the nervous system is so important in how we live and the role of stress on our health; however, by the end of the book he thought the magic was going to lie within the development of new drugs. I got so angry

---

1   "Why Zebras Don't Get Ulcers": Robert M. Sapolsky ISBN 0-7167-3210-6.

that I threw the book against the wall because he had gone this far and then decided to stay in the medical approach by adding another stressor with the use of chemicals (another drug). Really, that was the best he could come up with? He missed his own point!

Robert Sapolsky picked it up and he got it. The reason he called his book *Why Zebras Don't Get Ulcers*, is very interesting. Zebras are at the bottom end of the food chain; everybody is trying to eat them. They've got to stay in the alert response all the time and they're constantly scanning their environment for trouble. If they see or sense there is trouble happening, their nervous system goes into a full fight/flight response and they will run away. If they don't run fast enough, their worries are over. We know what the end result is there. If they do run fast enough and get to a place where they are safe, they stop and within 90 seconds their nervous system goes back to normal. You'd think they would have ulcers living a life like this, but because their system is so neuroplastic and adapts so beautifully, that is not what happens. The only time they do get ulcers, however, is if you lock them in a zoo. They can't run away. The stress never stops.

Adrenalin and Cortisol and the Immune System

Adrenalin and cortisol normally are secreted in response to a perceived threat in the environment. Adrenalin and cortisol are stress hormones secreted from the adrenal glands, which sit above the kidneys.

Adrenalin(Epinephrine) is a hormone produced by the medulla of the adrenal glands and is a crucial component of the fight-or-flight response of the sympathetic nervous system, which works to increase blood flow to the muscles and oxygen to the lungs. It has many functions in the body, regulating heart rate, blood vessel and air passage diameters, and metabolic shifts, all of which influence the immune system function.

Cortisol release is controlled by the hypothalamus, a part of the brain that in turn activates the pituitary gland, which activates the adrenal cortex to produce cortisol. Cortisol activates anti-stress and anti-inflammatory pathways. Though both chemicals are stress hormones, adrenalin and cortisol have different roles. Cortisol stimulates the liver and pancreas, which increases glucose levels available for muscles to use. It also temporarily inhibits other systems of the body, including digestion, growth, reproduction and the immune system.

Stress and Cholesterol

These two hormones, adrenalin and cortisol, trigger the production of cholesterol. Stressful situations create the demand for more energy. Cortisol produces more sugar in order to provide the body with instant energy. Continued stress produces high sugar levels that often are not used up by the body and eventually are converted to fatty acids and cholesterol. Stress also can push people toward unhealthy eating habits and lifestyles: smoking, drinking and eating a diet that contributes to high cholesterol. Cholesterol deposits start accumulating in the walls of arteries and other organs.

Although we are led to believe that cholesterol is a fat, it's more like an alcohol but it doesn't act like one. The highest percentage of cholesterol is found in the brain and nerve system, demonstrating it is a necessity for normal mental and brain function and activity. Cholesterol is also necessary for every cell in the body as it waterproofs the cell membranes. Cholesterol is made by all cells, however majority of our cholesterol is made by the liver. Less than 50% of the cholesterol we consume is actually absorbed.

The genders, male and female, are equally affected by stress when it comes to cholesterol production. The stress responses are cumulative and previous response patterns increase the amount of cholesterol production as new stressors are brought to life.[2] We now know, the higher the stress or longer duration the stress, the higher the level of Low Density Lipoprotein (LDL -the bad cholesterol). LDL is produced by the liver to act as a carrier of cholesterol.

However, there is another factor involved in arterial plaque

---

2 Mental stress raises cholesterol levels in healthy adults - Pam Willenzpwillenz@apa.org, American Psychological Associationhttp://www.apa.org -23 Nov 2005 - 13:00 PDT

According to researchers at Duke University, as a result of the stress/inflammation link, stress hormones stimulate the immune system to release inflammatory chemicals.[3] This stress response is now the primary factor in arterial plaque formation -so neurological stress responses play a much bigger factor in cardiovascular health than diet.

The foundational cause of arterial plaque is the perception of danger and a possible bleed injury. The brain does a defense response by releasing sticky platelets that are designed to form blood clots and stop a bleed out. The brain registers any threat (stressor) as a need for a fight/flight reaction and a potential bleed situation. The problem is that when no bleed takes place, the body has these very sticky platelets floating around in the blood vessel looking for some place to build a clot. Any rough area on a vessel wall or bifurcation (blood vessel division) provides an opportunity for them to attach. The problem is not so much cholesterol build up but is really the state of sustained stress responses. Drugs such as Lipitor reduce the so called bad cholesterol but research shows that the cholesterol drugs have little to no effect on the incidence of cardiovascular challenges. Basically, when it comes to the immune responses, including the production of adrenalin and cortisol, the role of stress is a much bigger health concern than diet.

---

3   "Beyond Cholesterol" -by Judith Mandelbaum-Schmid in Body and Soul, July/August 2004

Chapter 9-Things to Consider

☞ Stress is more than just feeling overwhelmed!

☞ Stress can be created by a belief that isn't real or truthful.

☞ There are different types of stress responses.

☞ Every system of the body is affected by stress.

☞ The role of stress in illness was researched in the 1960s but was not addressed until the 1990s.

☞ The ability to recover from stress is a key factor in health.

☞ Inflammation is a first level stress response and is controlled by the nervous system.

☞ Arterial plaque is not a high cholesterol problem; it is a stress response problem.

CHAPTER

TEN

What does the body do to react to stress?

Chapter 10.
What does the body do to react to stress?
Alert Response Mechanism (ARM)

When you put your body under stress, what is your body telling you? The information comes in as a warning. There are two different levels to this. There is a level called the Alert Response Mechanism[1] (ARM), which is the first stage of threat or early stress response --women are better at this than men. The world tends to be a bit more dangerous for women than men, so they're much more aware of their environment and what's going on around them than men tend to be.

Not only that, women tend to use both hemispheres of their brain. They have a larger corpus callosum, the part of the brain that transfers information back and forth between both left and right hemispheres. The corpus callosum[2,3,4] of men are a little smaller and men tend to be more left hemisphere dominate. So here is what is important about this information.

This alert response mechanism says there is something going on around you that's not right. You don't know what it is, but you pick up on it and you respond to it. Probably the best way to describe this is to visualize deer in a field. The deer are eating the grass when all of a sudden they stop, they look up and they freeze. There is a neurological response going on. They sense that there is something not right. When they freeze like that, their respiration literally stops, heart slows down, pupils dilate, hearing and smell increase and the ability of the eyes to pick up motion is focused on. We have cells in our brain that automatically register motion and will direct our attention to the motion[5].

This action is a protective measurement that's already built into the brain. The brain knows that survival depends on being alert even during a relaxed period. What happens if the deer see there is something dangerous going on, such as a pack of wolves coming out of the woods? They kick into full fight/flight mechanism and off they go. We will go into more detail about the fight/flight response in Chapter 14. If the deer don't see anything, they immediately return to normal and go back to eating grass. We have the same ability to return to normal or ideal. All living things have the same ability because a balanced system (homeostasis) is the key factor in life. ARM is the first level of sensory response to a perceived threat.

The brain cannot tell the difference between a real threat and perceived threat. As our life becomes surrounded by information overload, erratic actions, constant noise and challenged nutrition, the brain's threat threshold is lowered. The alert response starts to engage more often.

We have this communication device called television that allows us to see worldwide crises, earthquakes in Japan, a nuclear accident in Japan, and tidal waves. Even though we can't do anything about it, we share in the stress and fear of it, the sadness of it all and it affects us like we were right there. So we're registering stress from all directions such as pollution in the air, bad foods, or driving your car down the road with crazy drivers around you. There is enough stress simply dealing with these issues, plus we have set ourselves into a time scheduling stress pattern. We have instant access to everybody now with smart cell phones. You can rarely get quiet time. And financial challenges in the last few years are large in everybody's mind when we keep hearing about unemployment and so on. The news media talk about 8 percent unemployment and make it sound stressful when it really means there is 92 percent employment. If we could look at it that way, it would release stress. However, that would not keep our attention and doesn't sell anything, so the news media continues to focus on the negative. Our systems say danger, danger and we're in trouble.

There is another factor to consider which is what I call the "Chicken Little Factor". This is about Chicken Little who ran around yelling that the sky was falling so many times that no one listened any more. Not even when it did fall. The ARM serves a purpose but with the constant overload in today's life styles, the beautiful warning system designed to protect us from harm becomes numb. We fail to recognize the potential of danger until it is too late. An example would be comparing city dwellers with the constant noise of city life to someone from a remote island. The sound of an approaching car means little to the city person but would put the island person on alert. Some islanders may become hyper alert and jump at every movement or sound until they are exhausted.

The enteric nervous system[6] of the "Gut" plays a role in the ARM response. It is the old part of our nervous system and has around 100 million neurons (nerve cells). When you get that "Gut Feeling", that is just your enteric nervous system telling you something is not right in paradise.

We are emotionally based beings with all of our experiences imprinted into our memory banks with an emotional attachment[7]. These emotions are the power behind who we are. Our doubts and fears are our history talking to us subconsciously and may carry real information or they may not be real. Many of our doubts and fears are based on perceptions of an event which may not be accurate but nevertheless are embedded into our subconscious and continue to create responses that do us harm.

You may think that all is well because from a conscious awareness, you don't feel stressed or worried, and you seem to have good energy. You are conscientious about your diet and exercise and your life style pattern is consistent. Assumption: you are well and in good health.

Until just recently we have not been able to look into the subconscious workings of the nervous system to see if all you have assumed is true. We have had to wait for a symptom to appear to show that your body function has been disrupted.

This is the reason that most of the health professions have to rely on signs and symptoms to judge the state of a person's health. While a little late to offer the best results, this method was the best they had to offer during the development of the practice of medicine.

Neuroscience today, along with the development of computer driven instruments, has allowed us to record neurological responses driven by the subconscious and then, based on the information provided, start care plans before the system damage generates signs and symptoms of malfunction.

Chapter 10 - Things to Consider

☞ Alert Response Mechanism (ARM) is the first level of stress response.

☞ We have two brains in the form of left and right hemispheres.

☞ The hemispheres talk to one another.

☞ We have cells in the brain that detect motion.

☞ There are levels beyond the five senses that are sensory in nature.

☞ As stress increases, do trigger thresholds lower?

☞ Challenging information will create a response whether or not it directly involves you.

☞ The news media can create a dynamic effect on your stress responses.

References

1. "Alert Response Mechanism

2. "Characterization of sexual dimorphism in the human corpus callosum". ^ Dubb A, Gur R, Avants B, Gee J (2003). Neuroimage 20 (1): 512–9. doi:10.1016/S1053-8119(03)00313-6. PMID 14527611.

3. "Effects of handedness and gender on macro-and microstructure of the corpus callosum and its subregions: a combined high-resolution and diffusion-tensor MRI study". ^ Westerhausen R, Kreuder F, Dos Santos Sequeira S et al. (2004). Cognitive Brain Research 21 (3): 418–26. doi:10.1016/j.cogbrainres.2004.07.002. PMID 15511657.

4."Sex differences in the human corpus callosum: diffusion tensor imaging study". ^ Shin YW, Kim DJ, Ha TH et al. (2005). NeuroReport 16 (8): 795–8. doi:10.1097/00001756-200505310-00003. PMID 15891572.

5. "Neurons that detect motion rapidly switch between modes of data collection." The Salk Institute for Biological Studies in La Jolla, California, February 28, 2007

6. "The Abdominal Brain and Enteric Nervous System", David L. McMillin, M.A., Douglas G. Richards, Ph.D., Eric A. Mein, M.D., Carl D. Nelson, D.C. Meridian Institute Virginia Beach, VA 23454

7. "Long-term potentiation in the amygdala: a mechanism for emotional learning and memory". Maren S.Trends Neurosci. 1999 Dec;22(12):561-7. Review

C H A P T E R
E L E V E N

Your Life – A Drama Worth Living

Chapter 11.
Your Life – A Drama Worth Living
The Role of Stress Reponses

Stress is a fact of life! The real role of the stress response is survival. The collective knowledge of the cells of the body is geared toward survival. As the body is a collection of cells organized into organs and then systems, there needs to be a central organizing authority to orchestrate the complexities of a harmonious expression of life. The body is called a *closed loop system,* which means that the systems are dependent on each other to maintain a balance. An imbalance in any of the systems will affect other systems and will eventually lead to sickness and death. Any threat or stress not countered ideally will create an imbalance or anything less than an ideal recovery will reduce the survival value of the individual.

Stressors in moderation are, in reality, good for our systems. Even exercise is a stressor. Without it, muscle tone decreases and we lose power and mobility. Gravity helps our bones retain their strength. Our nervous system has developed a variety of responses to stressors that will provide a better ability to survive environmental challenges. These challenges can range from a perceived threat to an outright life-threatening event. Even a subconscious concept of a threat will be registered and the neurophysiology will act accordingly. For example: if as a child an adult was attacked by a dog and later on in life sees a dog similar to the one that attacked, the subconscious mind will trigger a stressful fear response. This will happen even though the adult knows they are safe from an attack. The subconscious will remember the danger and there will be changes in the neurophysiology of the body.

Here is the catch – it is not so much a matter of stressors or the stress response being the only culprits here, but your ability to recover from the experience also matters[1]. The ideal goal is for your body to regain a normal balance within your neurological function. Blood pres-

1   Stressed or stressed out: What is the difference?Bruce S. McEwen, J Psychiatry Neurosci. 2005 September; 30(5): 315–318. PMCID: PMC1197275

sure must return to ideal, hand temperature warms up, heart rate slows down, and respiration becomes slow and regular. Internally the stress response chemicals such as cortisol and adrenalin return to normal levels. Insulin and blood sugar levels return to normal. The body runs these systems innately, which means there is an inborn knowledge (innate) in each call, organ and system that knows how and when to act.

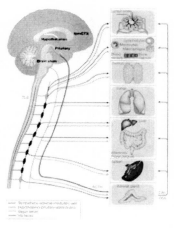

If this does not happen, then we have a problem and systems will start to break down because they are not designed to maintain a constant stress response activity level. If the body remains in the stress response state (even at a low level) over time there is a price to be paid. Remember the role of the immune system and its relationship to the nervous system? A prolonged level of a stress response state shuts down the immune response[2]!

The end result of a prolonged stress response and the most important factor for your good health lies in the effect it has on the great guardian, the immune system. Once the stress influence has damaged the relationship between the nervous system and the immune system, an individual is in grave (great choice of words) danger.

In the past 20 years, the field of psychoneuroimmunology[3] has demonstrated major connections between the stress pathways and the immune system. There are interactive two way connections between the nervous system, the endocrine system, and the immune system.

2   Protective and Damaging effects of stress mediators. McEwan BS., New England Journal of Medicine. 1983;338(3):171-179

3   Psychoneuroimmunology - (PNI), is a relatively recent branch of science that enforces beliefs that physicians have held for many centuries, perhaps well before the times of the ancient Greeks. The premise is that a patient's mental state influences diseases and healing. Specifically, PNI studies the connection between the brain and the immune system.The term psychoneuroimmunology was coined by Robert Ader, a researcher in the Department of Psychiatry at the University of Rochester Medical Center in Rochester, New York. In the 1970s, studies by Ader and other researchers opened up new understandings of how experiences such as stress and anxiety can affect a person's immune system.

These stress pathways[4] include: the Hypothalmo-pituitarymedulla (HPA) Axis; the Sympathetic-Adrenal-Medulla (SNS) Axis and the Vagus Nerve (PNS). The pathways have a direct and powerful effect on the immune system. The immune system has an innate or natural immune response (genetic patterns) and an adaptive immune response (experienced).

The immune system is a collection of billions of cells that travel through the bloodstream. They move in and out of tissues and organs, defending the body against foreign bodies (antigens) such as bacteria, viruses and cancerous cells.

Components of the Innate Immune system:

- Anatomical Barriers (mucous membrane)

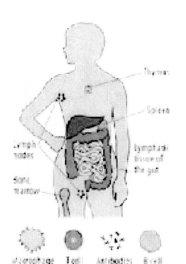

- Lymphatic system

- Phagocytosis

- Inflammation (Mast cells)

Natural Killer Cells:

Neutraphils

Monocytes

Molecules:

Complement proteins

Acute phase proteins

---

4   Stress, Endocrine Physiology and Pathophysiology - Eva Kassi, MD, Assistant Professor, Laboratory of Biological Chemistry, Medical School, University of Athens, - Constantine Tsigos, MD, Department of Endocrinology, HYGEIA Hospital, Athens, Greece - IoannisKyrou, MD, WISDEM, University Hospital Coventry and Warwickshire, Clinical Sciences Research Institute, Warwick Medical School, University of Warwick, Coventry - George P. Chrousos, MD, MACP, FRCP, Professor and Chairman, First Dept of Pediatrics Chief, Division of Endocrinology, Metabolism and Diabetes, University of Athens Medical School, Children's Hospital Aghia Sophia, Athens, Updated: June 1, 2012

Stress Facts

Stress is linked to: headaches, infectious illness (e.g. flu), cardiovascular disease, diabetes, asthma, gastric ulcers, chronic fatigue syndrome, cancer, irritable bowel syndrome, and more.

Stress can also have an indirect effect on the immune system, as a person may use unhealthy behavioral coping strategies to reduce their stress, such as drinking and smoking.

The stress hormone corticosteroid can suppress the effectiveness of the immune system (e.g. lowers the number of lymphocytes). If the production of cortisol is prolonged the immune system starts acting on its own.

When we're stressed, the immune system's ability to fight off antigens is reduced. That is why we are more susceptible to infections.

The main types of immune cells are white blood cells. There are two types of white blood cells – lymphocytes and phagocytes.

T cells - if the invader gets inside a cell, these (T cells) lock on to the infected cell, multiply and destroy it.

B cells- produce antibodies that are released into the fluid surrounding the body's cells to destroy the invading viruses and bacteria.

Things to Consider

☞ The body's systems depend on each other to function in harmony.

☞ There is an inborn knowledge (innate) in each cell, organ and system of the body.

☞ There is good stress and bad stress.

☞ Past events set up future stress response patterns.

☞ Prolonged stress has a direct effect on the immune response.

☞ As we now know the stress pathways, we can test them to learn how they are working.

☞ The effect of our stress response pattern involves many other systems of the body.

CHAPTER
TWELVE

The Immune Adaptive Group

Chapter 12.

The Immune Adaptive Group

The Action of the Adaptive Immune System

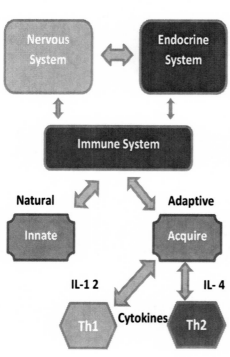

The previous chapter demonstrates that our stress response and stress recovery patterns are critical to understanding why our immune system is not functioning correctly. Have you noticed that there has been an increase of people with cancer; auto immune system diseases are growing at a rate of 23%[1] and that there is an increasing number of crazy allergic reactions to all sorts of items? Examples of autoimmune disorders include rheumatoid arthritis, multiple sclerosis, juvenile diabetes, cardiomyopathy, antiphospholipid syndrome, Guillain-Barré syndrome, Crohn's disease, Graves' disease, Sjogren's syndrome, alopecia, myasthenia gravis, lupus erythematosus, chronic fatigue syndrome and psoriasis. To make sense of this we need to look a little deeper into what happens with this breakdown between the brain and the immune system. We have two parts to the immune system: one being, the *natural* or *innate* division and the other the *adaptive* or *acquired* division. The innate portion comes from our genetic patterns while the acquired comes from exposure to immune challenges. Breast feeding[2] allows the infant to acquire a strong immune system by passing on the mother's well developed adaptive immune defenses.

Stress challenges to the nervous system directly affect the immune function and create a breakdown in the acquired division. The breakdown affects the action of immune development and involves complex activity which includes interleukin and cytokines. The important step here is the effect it has on the immune system stem cell development. Stem cells are cells that can change their function as they develop.[3] The immune adaptive group involves the formation of immune cells produced by the influence of cytokines (a protein released by cells that has a specific effect on the behavior of cells called T Helper cells, named Th1 and Th2). Maintaining a balance between Th1 and Th2 is critical for good immune system function. A decrease in cellular protection of Th1 stem cells leads to the formation of cellular immunity breakdown and mutations (such as cancer) while an increase of the Th2 stem cells that control humoral (general body) immunity leads to increased sensitivities to chemical agents, which leads to an increase in health challenges such as asthma and allergies. As we now look at our high stress lifestyles, we can begin to understand the exponential increase in cancers, hyper-sensitivities to nuts, other foods or chemicals and the exponential growth of auto¬immune system diseases of which the incidence in women is 75 percent higher than men.[4] Research on the brain and its function continues to reveal a new understanding of the cause of disease and illness.

Stress also decreases the production and action of the innate factors of the immune response.

As we now have an explanation of the role of the brain and the nervous system in relation to immune system activity, any brain injury will have a serious direct effect on the state of health for the individual.

We tend to view the term brain injury as a massive trauma, but with the above information we need to rethink the term. Any level of altered brain activity (abnormal pattern) is in fact a brain injury. The only difference is that the low level abnormal pattern is covert (unnoticed) in nature but has the same outcome over time. It will interfere with the immune system and create the shift to the right in cytokine production and therefore the Th1-Th2 relationship. When you add the altered brain function and the distorted messages being sent to the other body systems, we can begin to see how this new perspective on the cause of disease is rapidly gaining acceptance throughout the health professions.

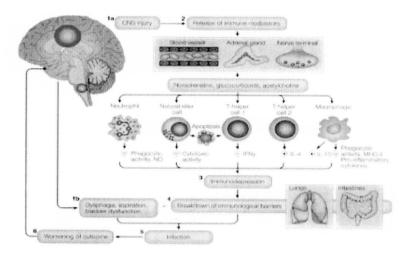

The chart shows the effects of brain injury and the immune response.

We are now beginning to see articles and papers on the effects of stress on every aspect of health concerns. Dentists are talking about the effects of stress on teeth and decay[5]. Prestigious medical schools such as: Stanford, Yale, Harvard, Duke, Johns Hopkins and Northwestern have recently published research that is changing the way doctors will treat pain or dysfunction. Chronic pain and dysfunction are now also seen as disorders of the brain and nerve system, not just the spine, joints or muscles. The research also states that the best treatments are the least invasive, don't involve surgery, address the injured spine, joints, or muscles and also address the painful or disruptive nerve signals in the brain The brain is the central organizing system of the body that controls all of the other systems.

The brain has the ability to receive information from the environment, design appropriate responses within the body then return to an ideal balance once the response has done its job. Homeostasis is the term that has been used in the past for this adaptive response. Homeostasis suggests a static balancing within the systems. Today we know this balance to be an active adaptive balance that deals with neurological control including relaxation, alert response, fight/flight action and most importantly recovery or a return to ideal balance. When the brain becomes impaired, when it becomes over stimulated, it loses the ability to keep itself regulated. It loses the ability of neuroplasticity, which is the ability to respond and adapt to the environment in the most ideal way.

This loss of neuroplasticity creates inappropriate patterns of response. The brain's processing resources start to become overloaded and you get inappropriate responses[6]. The inappropriate responses to stressors can be varied. It can be that you don't respond correctly to the stressor or you don't recover from the stressor. One of the key factors in all of this is recovery ability. Within 90 seconds after the stressor, your body should be able to get back down to ideal limits, which are the responses we look for when we're talking about stress.

Chapter 12 - Things to Consider

☞ List 5 stressors in your life of which you are aware.

☞ How long have you been aware of these?

☞ Have you noticed a health challenge when these stressors increase?

☞ Did you know there was a direct relationship between stress and autoimmune disorders?

☞ Concussion at any level is a traumatic brain injury and is cumulative in nature.

☞ Women are 75 percent more likely to develop an autoimmune system disorder.

References

1. "The Autoimmune Epidemic" by Donna Jackson Nakazawa, Publisher: Touchstone; 1 edition (February 5, 2008)ISBN-10: 0743277759 ISBN-13: 978-0743277754

2. Breastfeeding Benefits Your Baby's Immune System - healthychildren. org - American Academy of Pediatrics

3. A Primer on Stem Cells - by Lucie Bruijn, PhD, The ALS Association's Senior Vice President of Research and Development American Autoimmune Related Diseases Association (http://www. aarda.org).

4. Researchers look at causes of autoimmune diseases - By Jamie Lampros Standard-Examiner correspondent Sat, 07/14/2012 - 9:19pm

5. Chart - Meisel et al., Nature Rev. Neurosci. 6:775-786, 2005

6. Stress can contribute to poor oral health - Scott Gargan, Staff Writer - Published 12:25 p.m., Wednesday, February 23, 2011   OTHER LIVING - http://www.stamfordadvocate.com/health/article/Stress-can-contribute-to-poor-oral-health-1026740.php#ixzz2BSu951GS

7. Brain Economics: - Housekeeping Routines in the Brain - Proefschrift ter verkrijging van het doctoraat in de Medische Wetenschappen aan de Rijksuniversiteit Groningen op gezag van de Rector Magnificus, dr. F. Zwarts, in het openbaar te verdedigen op maandag 5 oktober 2009 om 14.45 uur door Paolo Toffanin geboren op 12 maart 1979 te Sandrigo, Itali¨e Promotores : Prof. dr. A. Johnson Prof. dr. R. de Jong Prof. dr. G.J. ter Horst Copromotor : Dr. S. Martens Beoordelingscommissie : Prof. dr. M. Eimer Prof. dr. B. Hommel Prof. dr. N.M. Maurits ISBN (boek): 978-90-367-3979-5   ISBN (digitaal): 978-90-367-3978-8

C H A P T E R
T H I R T E E N

Understanding Stress - The Stress Response

Chapter 13.

Understanding Stress - The Stress Response

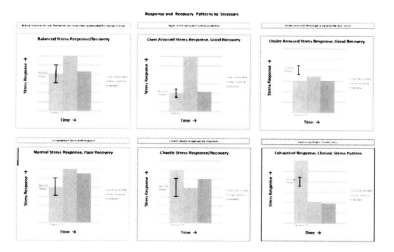

There are 6 different states of Stress Reponses patterns

Light Grey - Normal Neurophysiological response
Middle Grey- Stressor responses
Dark Grey – Recovery

1. **Top left** -Ideal response–a neurological state that is alert, relaxed; then an acute response to a stressor; followed by a return to the ready relaxed state.

2. **Center top** - The Over-aroused Response –Alert relaxed, ready; then to an over reacted neurological response; with a return to the ready relaxed state.

3. **Top right** -The Under-aroused Response – impaired ready; then to an impaired stress response; back to impaired ready.

4. **Bottom left** - The Poor Recovery Response -alert ready;then to acute response to a stressor; with impaired recovery. This loss of recovery is accumulative in nature and moves the system into

imbalance.

5. **Bottom middle** - Chaotic Response – over sensitive ready state, then to a collapsed response; some recovery. The added stressor overloads the response as the processing resources of the brain begin to malfunction. Inappropriate output from the brain creates further imbalance in the body system and therefore raises the level of stressors. This leads to an exhausted nervous system.

6. **Bottom right** - Exhausted Nervous System — over sensitive ready state; then to a collapsed response; with no recovery. This stage is a chronic level response and includes an exhausted immune system as well. The over sensitive ready state has the immune system so overloaded with threat messages that it has gone into total defense and now attacks everything it perceives as a threat. The exhausted state is the highest level of the brain's impaired ability to regulate itself as it involves a total breakdown of communication between the endocrine, immune and central organization authority–the brain.

How did you develop the stress response pattern?

These stress response patterns are created by two factors: one being the genetic predisposition and the second being the result of your experiences. There is still much discussion regarding the role of genetic expression in so far as genes don't turn themselves on and are influenced by the environment. The role they play in the development of a pattern ranges from 20 to 50 percent according to the latest research[1].

This suggests the response patterns we have are primarily a result of our perception of stressors in our life and how we have dealt with them over time.

The misconception is that we are stuck with these patterns, whether genetic or experience based. We are not, and we can learn how to improve these patterns.

---

1   Chronic Stress May Cause Long-Lasting Epigenetic Changes - 09/15/2010 -Release Date: 09/15/2010 http://www.hopkinsmedicine.org/psychiatry/expert_team/faculty/P/Potash.html

The new debate is about how the ability of the brain to create new neural pathways influences our genetic innate prewiring[2]. The key is the application of appropriate intervention and retraining to build the new pathways. Without this, the prewiring will dominate.

Chapter 13 – Things to Consider

☞ Into which stress response group do you think you fit?

☞ What does this mean to your health?

☞ How long has this been your pattern?

☞ What would your life be like if you could improve your response pattern?

☞ While we must deal with "stressors" every day, the real challenge is, "Are you able to recover from the stress?"

☞ Can you place someone you know (family member, friend, co-worker) into one of the patterns?

2   Metabolite Abnormalities in Fibromyalgia: Correlation With Clinical Features. P. Wood, C. Ledbetter, M. Glabus, L. Broadwell, J. Patterson 2nd. Hippocampal The Journal of Pain, 2008; DOI: 10.1016/j.jpain.2008.07.003

CHAPTER

FOURTEEN

Understanding Stress - The Stress Response

Chapter 14.
What is "Survival Value"?

B.J. Palmer (Developer of Chiropractic) was talking with one of his dear friends, a well-known philosopher, Elbert Hubbard. They were having a discussion around a table and B.J. asked his friend what he thought were the most important words in the English language. Elbert Hubbard[1] thought about it and answered, "Survival value." Survival value means that the most valuable thing in the whole world for any living creature is to be able to survive. Anything you do that creates an increase in your ability to survive in your environment adds to that value. So you have longevity if you have good survival value. You have good health: that means good survival value. A balanced nervous system is good survival value. Good nutrition: good survival value. You need to consider all these things to see how you can apply it to your life. By contrast: Cigarette smoking? - Poor survival value. Bad nutrition: poor survival value. Everything you do to add to your survival value is going to add to the quality of your life and the longevity of your life.

What Influences Survival Value?

What is your body telling you under stress? The first information that comes in is a warning. We discussed the Alert Response Mechanism (ARM) in Chapter 10. The next stress response is the fight/flight response mechanism. There are several physiological responses that engage during fight/flight response and every response is based on the need to survive in a short time threat period. Every physiological action during the fight/flight response reaction is based on improving the chances of survival, but in order to do so, the ideal balance of the system gets disrupted. We have adrenalin and cortisol being produced

---

1   Elbert Green Hubbard (June 19, 1856 – May 7, 1915) was an American writer, publisher, artist, and philosopher. Raised in Hudson, Illinois, he met early success as a traveling salesman with the Larkin soap company. Today Hubbard is mostly known as the founder of the Roycroft artisan community in East Aurora, New York, an influential exponent of the Arts and Crafts Movement. Among his many publications were the nine-volume work Little Journeys to the Homes of the Great and the short story A Message to Garcia. He and his second wife, Alice Moore Hubbard, died aboard the RMS Lusitania, which was sunk by a German submarine off the coast of Ireland on May 7, 1915.

at a very high rate for the fight or flight. These two hormones are designed to be used in short duration and limited amounts. If production is prolonged they have devastating effects on all the body's systems.[2]

The Fight /Flight responses

One of the F/F responses is cold hands and feet. Why does that happen? It happens because the brain or *innate intelligence* says I need blood to go to the big muscles so that I can run fast or have good muscle activity to fight. So I'm going to pull blood away from the extremities and bring it into the central core so I can oxygenate the blood and be able to get it going to the big muscles. The reduction of blood flow in the hands and feet makes them lose the heat from the blood supply.

The next thing that happens is that the hands become sweaty. If you've ever been in a high stress situation, you immediately notice you've got cold, clammy hands. The reason that your hands sweat is because fingerprints are good for gripping but work much better when they're damp. It's like when you lick your fingers to do a better job of turning the pages of a book. Automatically the body says, "If I'm going to fight, I have to be able to grab things. I want to be able to grab things the best way I can. I'm going to make my hands moist so that they'll stick."

Another stage of increased skin moisture during a stress response says, "I'm going to also make my body very slippery. I'm going to have that cold sweat on my body so that when people try to grab me they can't hang on." These are all self-protection mechanisms that the brain does automatically when it gets into a fight/flight or stressful situation.

Heart rate goes up so it can supply nutrition and oxygen and remove carbon dioxide from the body in a fight/flight situation. Your respiration is going to go up, for the same reason. Your liver and your pancreas are kicked into gear because that's where we develop the energy to run the systems. If we are running under a constant and chronic fight/flight pattern with high demands on the liver and pancreas, they will not be

---

2   "Why Zebras Don't Get Ulcers": Robert M. Sapolsky ISBN 0-7167-3210-6.

able to keep up and one of the results is Type 2 diabetes[3]. This health challenge is on a rampage in this country and it's all based on stress.

Remember, I also said nutrition can be a stress indicator. If you're eating poorly, you're going to be stressing the body which can lead to Type 2 diabetes as well. Even if we think we can control the information overflow consciously, the subconscious hears every word, sees every picture, smells, feels and tastes every event that affects us. It is called sensory input. All of our sensory input goes into the brain, gets attached to an emotion and then is transferred to the cortex for experience storage and reference information.

Stressors are normal in our life. We will experience alert and flight/fight responses throughout the day, and the nervous system has divisions that not only speed up the system to deal with the stress but also divisions to cool the body back to an ideal relaxed state.

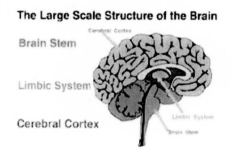

The Large Scale Structure of the Brain

Brain Stem

Limbic System

Cerebral Cortex

Now we're going to look at cortical activity and see what's going on in the cortex during stress responses. The cortex is a huge storage facility for our experiences, including our lessons in sight, sounds, taste, touch, smell, our doubts and fears all linked with an emotional attachment. It is our reference library. The cortex produces electrical energy of varying frequencies depending on the state of activity. These changes in frequencies during activity are called brain waves. We can divide the brain into two hemispheres, which is important, because they view the world differently[4].

The two hemispheres are linked together by a connection called the Corpus callosum and exchange information continually. If they're not working together we have an imbalance called brain *hemispheric-*

3 Stress - Living with Diabetes- American Diabetes Associationwww.diabetes.org › Complications

4 One skull + two brains = four objects in mind.ScienceDaily. Retrieved December 13 - Massachusetts Institute of Technology (2011, July 5).

ity, which adds to our stress response. Any level of interference to ideal cortical function will have dire consequences to other areas of the brain depending on the message from the cortex. One of the primary areas in constant communication with the cortex is the limbic system.

The limbic system is one of the oldest parts of the brain and controls a critical part of the nervous system called the *autonomic nervous system* (ANS). The ANS of the body is divided into the *sympathetic* --that's the one that goes into gear for us to run away from the bear that's chasing us or the flight/fight mechanism; and the other called the *parasympathetic*, which is the slowdown recovery relax mode. By using these two balancing parts, the limbic system controls things such as blood pressure, heart rate, respiration, muscle tone, hand temperature and skin conductance.

These physical responses are all ways of being able to see how your system is functioning when it comes to stress and the ability to recover, and we can even take a look at it from the different types of stressors. We have a stressor that's a cognitive stress. That's where you have to think. You have to engage the brain and engage the cortex and be able to come up with a solution to a problem, especially under pressure. Another one is the emotional stressor which is huge because that deals with a great deal of the subconscious mind and those patterns that could have been established when you were an infant, some of them even in utero. Then the last one is the physical stressor and how you respond to physical stressors, which can involve things such as muscle tone and what's going on with the way you breathe, your heart function and so on.

Stressors stimulate the sympathetic portion of the nervous system. Continual stress keeps the fight/flight state in place. This means that your nervous system is producing adrenalin and cortisol at a high rate with no relief. These hormones are known as the *killer cocktail* of the body[5]. They are the hormones responsible for the production of bad cholesterol, diabetes, heart disease and strokes, just to name a few.

---

5   The urban jungle's most feared killer - Coaching for Changewww.coachingforchange.co.za/_the_urban_jungles_most_feared_kill...

Chapter 14 – Things to Consider

☞ Did you ever think that all our actions and/or our environment create the need-to-survive response within the nervous system?

☞ Did you know that much of our body's responses to stress begins with information received below the conscious awareness level?

☞ Every action of the body's system is motivated by survival instincts, such as cold hands and cold sweat responses.

☞ Type 2 diabetes is a direct result of your system becoming burned out from stress overload over time.

☞ Are you beginning to see the role of stressors on our lives and the relationship to illness?

C H A P T E R
F I F T E E N

**How Will a New Understanding
of Stress Effects be Helpful?**

Chapter 15.

How Will a New Understanding of Stress Effects be Helpful?

There are two ways of looking at what's going on within the body during stress responses. One is the foundation for the typical method of health-care today. Up until now we tended to look at factors after the stress response has happened and think that is the result or symptom is the challenge--for instance head-aches.

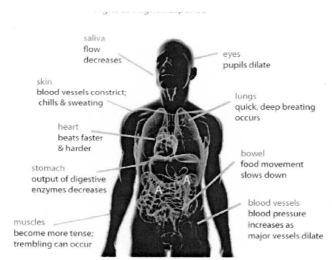

saliva flow decreases

eyes pupils dilate

skin blood vessels constrict; chills & sweating

lungs quick, deep breating occurs

heart beats faster & harder

bowel food movement slows down

stomach output of digestive enzymes decreases

blood vessels blood pressure increases as major vessels dilate

muscles become more tense; trembling can occur

What our sick care system generally does is to treat the head-ache instead of treating the less than ideal neurological response to the stressor that cre¬ated the headache. Now we need to understand how our stress challenges create a shift away from ideal neurological function, which leads to system breakdown, producing signs and symptoms and illness.

The stress response starts with sensory input that can be visual or auditory. It can be nutritional, or physical. It can be social or chemical. All of these factors are part of our intake through our sensory systems in order to register what's going on in our environment.

The gathered information is then fed into the brain, after which the brain takes a look at whether or not it has already had this experience. That's the function of the cortex of the brain.

The cortex stores our experiences and our memories with an emotional imprint. Think of the cortex of the brain as your personal library of experiences[1]. Most of these experiences, while you were very aware of the events as they happened, over time have become imprinted into your subconscious. Because of this, you are not aware that they control much of your life actions. To top all of this off, since we are human beings there is another factor to consider. One of the characteristics that make us unique is that we have this wonderful emotional overlay. The imprinting of our experiences is reinforced by an emotional attachment to the experience. The imprinted memory will be triggered into action, and here is the catch, whether at the conscious level or the subconscious level, by the emotional connection.

Let me give you an example.

Say you were attacked by a dog when you were young. That memory of terror imprinted into your subconscious so that whenever you see a dog of that type, you get a physical reaction even if the the dog is passive. Some of these memories can be imprinted as genetic patterns or even in utero[2,3], from a mother's experience during the pregnancy.

The emotional triggers use the senses to fire the response, so a trigger may be an odor such as fresh bread or smoke. Touch, taste, sight and sound or any combination are all foundations to start a retrieval of a memory. This will also start the emotional reaction attached to the memory, which may include hate, happiness, fear, hope, and/or

1   Learning and Memory - John H. Byrne, Ph.D., Department of Neurobiology and Anatomy, The UT Medical School at Houston

2   Fetus to Mom: You're Stressing Me Out! WebMD Featurewww.medicinenet.com ›women's health az list

3   The Womb, Your Mother, Yourself. Cancer, Heart Disease, Obesity, Depression, Scientists can now trace adult health to the nine months before birth by Annie Murphy Paul

sadness.

For example, those veterans suffering from war-related post traumatic stress disorder (PTSD) will respond to any noise that sounds like gunfire, and be immediately taken back into that fearful situation with all the emotions surrounding it.

As we go through life we continually experience new challenges and environments and with this continue to build new neural connections. The new pattern may connect with past experience patterns and carry with them the emotional overlay. Our belief system is based on these patterns and may or may not be accurate. The response to the emotional trigger is very real however, and the body will respond accordingly.

If the experience is recognized, it then knows what to do and sends a response down to the limbic system[4], which controls most of the body's basic functions and its responses to the messages from the cortex. Once the limbic system is kicked into gear, the defense mode is under way and the stress response goes into high gear.

Until recently our only recourse was to attempt to relax (whatever that meant) or take some medicine that would shut off the conscious awareness. The problem with the meds is that they didn't remove the stressor and the subconscious still had to deal with the challenge. To make matters worse, the drug soon became a stressor of a different source.

This begins to sound like a bleak picture so before you run out and buy a gun, which would make matters even worse, there is some good news to share about the ability to change your response patterns. You can change all your response patterns, up to and including your hard-

4   Limbic System: Amygdala - Anthony Wright, Ph.D., Department of Neurobiology and Anatomy, The UT Medical School at Houston

core brain wiring patterns. Even your genetic pattern can be changed.

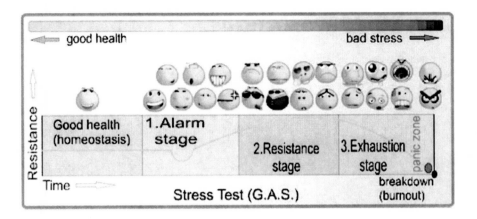

The first step is to recognize that you have stress patterns and how they affect your actions. As we have stated, many of these responses are at the subconscious level so while you may think you are fine, the truth may not support your belief. In fact we continue to see people with terrible physiological responses who think they are just fine. "De-Nile" isn't just a river in Egypt! The problem is that they don't act until symptoms appear and often times it can be fatal.

As we all have stress in our lives, we can relate to some of the early signs of fear, anxiety, and perhaps even some level of physical challenge. As time goes by, we build our individual patterns that we began to accept as normal. A great example of this is someone who has cold hands and when this is addressed they respond with, "Yes, but they are always cold." Once you understand that some of your patterns are outside the ideal, we can then address those issues before the challenge does permanent damage.

Chapter 15 -Things to consider

☞ Do you have past experiences that affect how you react today?

☞ Can you recognize that these challenges are silent stressors?

☞ Can you determine if you have any patterns that are outside of ideal?

☞ Are there any responses of which you are aware that were set by an event in your past?

☞ Does this help you to understand the origin of some of your health challenges?

CHAPTER
SIXTEEN

How Stress Affects Your Health--
and What You Can Do About it.

Chapter 16.

How Stress Affects Your Health--and What You Can Do About it.

The brain has this inborn ability to determine what it needs to do to protect itself to the point where it will sacrifice other parts of the body to save itself.

Here is a nightmare scenario. You are caught in an uprising and someone comes at you with a machete. As they swing it at you, you put your arm up to protect yourself. You know you're going to lose that arm but the brain doesn't care. The brain says, "I'm the most important part of the whole system. You can live without an arm but you can't live with-out me", That goes for the rest of the body. The brain will do what it needs to do to protect itself regardless of damage to any other part of the body. The processing resources (areas designed for specific functions) of the brain are set up on a priority basis. Along with this are

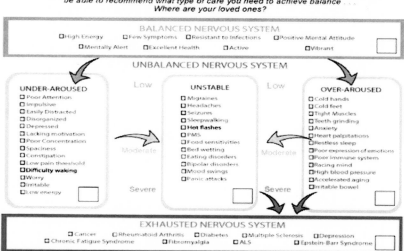

levels of stress responses based on intensity and duration of the stressor. That's why we have reactions such as high blood pressure and high heart rate, knowing full well that if you have high blood pressure and high heart rate over a period of time it's going to kill you. But the brain says, "That's not my concern at this moment. My concern is I need to respond to what's going on in the environment. If that means I have to run away or pump more blood to an area or speed up the heart, I'm going to do that." If the patterns are continually reinforced they become hard wired (neuronal connections) and create a fixed neurological pattern. These fixed neurological patterns present as over aroused, under aroused, unstable, or exhausted[1].

What is an over-aroused nervous system?

We can look at the cortical activity in the brain to see if it is stuck in high gear which would show up in an EEG as too much Beta brain wave activity. This is a frequency designed for fight/flight, or an alert response, which demands a huge amount of energy, so healing and/or recovery are not able to take place. All the energy of the nervous system is being spent in protection. This state is called an over-aroused nervous system. The signs and symptoms of an over-aroused system are high blood pressure, high heart rate, lots of adrenalin, lots of cortisol, cold hands, and high respiration rate to name a few (see chart). We see the stress response manifesting physically and if it stays that way there are consequences. This fight/flight high Beta state was designed for short term duration and if maintained for a prolonged time period is extremely damaging to all systems. No recovery or healing is able to take place.

What is an under-aroused nervous system?

When cortical activity is stuck in low gear which would show up as too much Theta/Delta brain wave activity, we say that the system is under-aroused. Theta (light sleep) and Delta (deep sleep) are subconscious brain activity. Slow responses and lack of focus are part of this picture. Health challenges such as hypoglycemia, ADD, low blood pressure and constipation are examples (see chart). People with dominant Theta brain activity are basically sleep walking and will be limited in ability to exhibit quick clear thinking.

What is an unstable or bipolar nervous system?

This level of neurological dysfunction shifts from over-arousal to under-arousal in an abstract time frame. This is an unstable system where one day it may react in an over-aroused state and the next day it may be

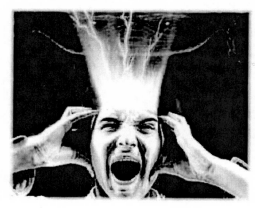

under-aroused. It could shift throughout the day without apparent cause. The unstable system is a sign that the neuroplasticity and control systems have become unstable and chaotic. If that continues it can lead to what we call an exhausted nervous system. Signs and symptoms of both over and under-aroused responses can be evidenced plus more severe challenges such as migraines, PMS and/or mood swings.

What is an exhausted nervous system?

The exhausted nervous system is showing up on tests more these days because we live in this highly stressful climate. In the exhausted nervous system, we see that systems are so disrupted that the immune system becomes overly distorted with inappropriate neurological information so that it can't respond correctly. The immune system is so overloaded that it thinks everything is an enemy and literally starts to attack everything.

This is where the autoimmune system disorders come into play. The autoimmune system disorders are growing exponentially and they include things such as Epstein-Barr, fibromyalgia, cancer, ALS, and multiple sclerosis to name a few. (see chart) All these challenges are the conditions in which the system literally has turned on itself, which is just a sign of that system being so disrupted that it's no longer able to determine what's right and what's wrong. This is a serious health challenge

While we have been trained to think of loss of health as some outside process, the truth is the opposite. All disease is a result of a failure of internal function. That could be a failure of the immune system to cope with an invading bacteria or virus, or a failure of the system to adapt or recover from stress factors. These factors include nutrition, physical injury, conditioning, mental issues, genetic weakness and the one which no one can avoid time.

Chapter 16 - Things to Consider

☞ Did you ever realize the hierarchy of the brain in self-defense?

☞ Our neurological patterns are developed through our stress responses.

☞ When the nervous system loses the ability to adapt and recover, the system becomes unbalanced.

☞ When the system is unbalanced it disrupts the function of the body.

☞ Symptoms are the only way the body can tell you something is wrong.

☞ Which do you think is better - Treating the symptoms or correcting the cause?

Reference

1. EEG Neurofeedback: A Generalized Approach to Neuroregulation – Siegfried Othmer, Susan Othmer and David Kaiser

CHAPTER
SEVENTEEN

**Understanding the Body's
Self Correction.**

Chapter 17.

Understanding the Body's Self Correction.

The first point to be considered here is that the body actually has the ability to self-correct. We have always recognized that the body indeed has a self-correcting, self-healing capability but at the same time understand that there is a limit to these actions. These two concepts seem to be contradictory in nature. How can they both exist? It is not unlike a truck. When new, the truck can withstand a lot of abuse but as the wear and tear accumulates, the parts wear out. If the abuse continues, breakdowns occur more frequently. Even though the body is a living adaptable system, it too has limits of recovery that are affected by time and damage.

When we look at how the body responds and adapts, processes food, defends itself, converts air to usable oxygen, eliminates waste, reproduces, regulates heat and cold, plus all the other functions at the same time, we begin to understand the complexity of life itself. The body is called a "closed loop system", which means that all the functions are related to one another and must remain in harmonic balance to function ideally. This is the job of the central nervous system (CNS), or as I like to call it - the central organizing authority. Its job is to maintain the harmonic balance throughout all the systems while continually gathering new information which will improve survival. The more you learn about the brain, the more you will be amazed at all it does. However, along with this knowledge you will also realize that stressors in our life interfere with its ideal function.

The concept of neurological self-correction is good to a point. Given the opportunity, the brain will always try to move systems back toward a balanced state, but that doesn't always work. As life stressors have a constant effect on nervous system function, the system builds neurological patterns of responses. These patterns become hard wired patterns based on the brain neuronal (brain cell) connections and are part of long term memory. While these patterns may be appropriate for short term responses, the fact that the stressors are constant creates a dilemma for the entire system. The high level of threat overloads the system and the ability to recover is lost. We like to think that the body has the ability to self-correct and self-heal which is true to a point, but once the nervous system has been pushed to the point of defense for survival, the ability to heal is compromised. All responses are defensive in nature. Add drugs into the mix and you introduce additional chemical stressors. A drug is given that is specific for one particular symptom but the secondary effects of that drug unbalance other systems. This explains why the average American is on five to seven different drugs by age fifty, and ten to twelve by age seventy. It is like "robbing Peter to pay Paul," except we know who is getting paid here.

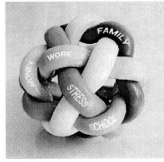

Today's lifestyle is one of constant stimulation. Television and radio, cell phones, noise, traffic, work demands and active children are all demands placed on our nervous system. We have even taken the concept of a quiet relaxing stroll and changed it to timed running with heart rate targets. Meals have become a timed event that we fit into our activities. In our search for pleasure we lost the reward of quiet non-structured relaxation. All of the rush, rush, needing to stay active and in touch with the world, has created havoc on our ability to recover. This state of high activity keeps our nervous system, our immune system and our endocrine system on constant alert status. The first level of response to an injury is an inflammatory reaction. The high stressor lifestyle hardwires the nervous system into an alert response so that we are held in a low level inflammatory state constantly[1].

Today's neuroscience is pointing in a completely different direction from the old days of medicine. Medicine continues to look at a bunch of signs and symptoms. Things are shifting today. Yesterday medicine was saying inflammation[2] is the crux of all this, but that inflammation is simply a normal response to injury. However, when you take a look at what controls the inflammation response, it is the central nervous system. In other words, the inflammatory response is a neurologically controlled response. This means that while inflammation is a normal first response to an injury, it has an ideal time frame. Research has shown that the initial inflammation response should last two to three days, and if it is still in action after five to seven days, the inflammation spreads to areas that were not part of the original injury. After ten to twelve days, if the inflammation has not reduced, the system starts to build scar tissue to stop the spread. This then indicates that there is a breakdown in the control system. These health challenges are actually challenged neurological function. The real problem in the loss of health lies within the brain's impaired ability to regulate itself. The loss of this ability leads to a breakdown in the closed loop system and the regulation of the body becomes unbalanced. Once the system is unbalanced, we lose the ability of self-correcting and self-healing. Our beautifully designed self-sustaining life force no longer exists and the only way we learn that we are in trouble is because now we start to develop symptoms.

By now you have probably noted that I continue to discuss the effects of stressors on brain function. The reason for this ongoing and somewhat repetitive dialog is due to the need to establish that what we have believed as health facts, such as bacteria and viruses being the cause of disease, or that any challenge to our health must be classified as a disease, are just plain and simply wrong.

It has been far too easy to turn any health challenge over to the medical community, let them tell you that you have "such and such" disease and therefore you need to take this medicine to be well. This has been our system for over a hundred years, so to create a shift in this thinking you need a lot of sound information to make better decisions about your health.

In fact the body *is* a self-healing self-maintaining being, which leaves us with the nagging question, why do some people get sick while others don't? Should we not all be able to maintain good health?

When we are all exposed to the same bacteria or virus and some get sick while others don't, it means that there is some other factor involved. It comes down to the loss of the body's ability to defend itself and in the worst scenario, lose the ability to self-heal. Once the system of self-maintenance has failed, then it is the ideal time for medical intervention, but not before as doing so only interfere with the body's ability to self-heal[4].

Chapte 17 - Things to Consider

Have you ever wondered how we stay healthy?

If everyone else was vaccinated and therefore is supposed to be immune, why the fuss about the people who are not vaccinated?

Why do some people in the same environment not catch a cold while others do?

What is a disease? Would we be better to think of it as dis-ease in the body's ability to function ideally?

Do we really need to be taking all the meds? And should we consider it normal to be on five to seven a day at age fifty?

What meds are you currently taking because of a problem caused by a previous med?

References

1, 2. How Stress Influences Disease: Study Reveals Inflammation as the Culprit - Science News - Apr. 2, 2012 - www.sciencedaily.com/releases/2012/04/120402162546.htm

3. Experimental Osteoarthritis in the Rabbit - Comparison of Different Periods of Repeated Immobilization Tapio Videman - Acta orthop. scand. 53, 339-347, 1982

4. The Epidemic of Overmedication - Use of multiple drugs, especially in older adults, can exacerbate ailments - By Siri Carpenter - www.msnbc.msn.com/id/27645077/ns/.../epidemic-overmedication/

CHAPTER
EIGHTEEN

**What is the Difference Between Acute Stress
and Chronic Stress?**

Chapter Eighteen

What is the Difference Between Acute Stress and Chronic Stress?

Acute Stress

We all have days in which we go through acute stress. Acute stress relates to something that has happened within the last 24 hours. It may be a car accident, or the water heater leaked, or perhaps you got a bill from the IRS. Acute stress can last from seconds to a few days. What happens with acute stress is that ideally you should go through the typical stress responses where your nervous system places the body into a high level of protection mode. All functions that are not directly related to protection are shut down. At the same time every function that will help you survive a crisis is totally engaged. As the focus has shifted to survival, the non-essential short term functions are dialed down. Fight/ flight responses are fast acting and they should recover within an hour. This describes an acute stress response. (See the initial stress response chart) This chart offers a compressed picture of the responses we have been explaining up to this point. It also offers a method of how to measure your level of stress response. Research over the years has been able to provide ideal ranges of responses for each of the categories listed[1].

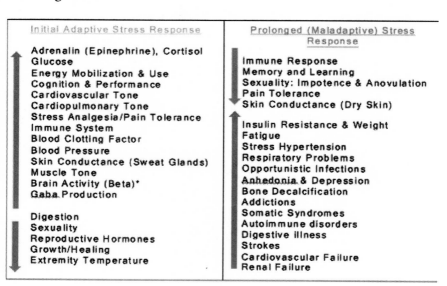

Initial Adaptive Stress Response	Prolonged (Maladaptive) Stress Response
Adrenalin (Epinephrine), Cortisol Glucose	Immune Response
Energy Mobilization & Use	Memory and Learning
Cognition & Performance	Sexuality: Impotence & Anovulation
Cardiovascular Tone	Pain Tolerance
Cardiopulmonary Tone	Skin Conductance (Dry Skin)
Stress Analgesia/Pain Tolerance	Insulin Resistance & Weight
Immune System	Fatigue
Blood Clotting Factor	Stress Hypertension
Blood Pressure	Respiratory Problems
Skin Conductance (Sweat Glands)	Opportunistic Infections
Muscle Tone	Anhedonia & Depression
Brain Activity (Beta)*	Bone Decalcification
Gaba Production	Addictions
	Somatic Syndromes
Digestion	Autoimmune disorders
Sexuality	Digestive illness
Reproductive Hormones	Strokes
Growth/Healing	Cardiovascular Failure
Extremity Temperature	Renal Failure

Chronic Stress

People don't realize that chronic stress is a real killer. Chronic stress is much more subtle. It is stress that has gone on for a long period of time, which can be weeks, months or years. It is something that has primarily happened to you, perhaps an experience that you can't let go of; or it is something in which the subconscious knows what was done was wrong and there is a huge emotional attachment. We start to see that there is a constant subconscious nagging going on with doubts and fears. These challenges are stored in Theta, the subconscious. These challenges are the "boogey men" that hide under the bed and it's the subconscious voice that talks to you when you have doubts and fears. Some of them may be based on the truth of some action in the past and some may be just an incorrect perception. These subconscious thoughts (the 80 to 90 percent of brain activity) force the brain into building your standard operating level, your stress response reaction and your recovery. We start to see life activities remaining consistently a challenge--one of the prime examples being *skin conductance.*

I previously wrote about how your hands get moist so you can grip when you come under stress. Well, it's not one of the critical life supports of stress. Having a heart that operates is a critical part. When you compare heart rate or respiratory rate to skin conductance, skin conductance is found lower on the scale of importance. What the system does under chronic stress is to take all its energy simply to keep going and to deal with things on a daily basis as well as this weight you're carrying on your back. Therefore, it will literally shut down the skin conductance in the hands, creating very dry hands which are no longer able to generate moisture because the brain shuts down that neurological response to be able to supply energy to other more critical areas. The typical response is to apply skin moisturizer which in the long view just shuts down the natural system even more. When you see this dry skin reaction, normally you see other areas that are really upset as well because very low skin conductance is a chronic stress level response.

At this point, we need to start looking into how best to deal with the stressors in your life. Research is now telling us that 95 percent of all illness is directly related to stress. The first step in your life will be to find some way to reduce the amount of stressors; easy to say but not so easy to do as life does go on and we can't just go back to the 60s attitude of let's just drop out. Steven Covey's book, *Seven Habits of Highly Effective People*, has a great chart on how to categorize daily events. It is a four part chart that puts daily tasks into perspective such as urgent and important versus not urgent but important. By following this chart, it will reduce a lot of unnecessary self-generated stress. The other side of this, however, is not as easy to handle. We will need to begin the process to change built in neurological responses that you have developed over years.

It is only in the last ten years that research into brain function has demonstrated that this is possible. Until recently we believed that the brain was set into patterns when we were young and also that there were no new brain cells developed after that stage. Oh how wrong we were about so much in our understanding about health, illness, disease and how we heal.

There are still some issues about health challenges we need to review, which are directly related to brain function, before we can begin to explain the way back to health. In the next few chapters we are going to look at the role of Attention Deficit Disorder (ADD), and its relationship to Post Traumatic Stress Disorder (PTSD), as well as the effects of stress over time; details of how to know when you are in a stress response, and a new approach toward how to change your reaction patterns and improve your life.

By now I hope that you have a better understanding of how and why your system weakens and that the responses you have are really self-induced, albeit, mostly at a subconscious level but nevertheless not created by some mystery invader.

Chapter 18 - Things to Consider

Stress is more than just a word.

Stress over time is the most serious threat to our health!

There are actions you can take that will not only reduce your stressors but will also change your current response patterns.

References

1. "Why Zebras Don't Get Ulcers": Robert M. Sapolsky ISBN 0-7167-3210-6.

CHAPTER
NINETEEN

How Does the Brain Actually Work?

Chapter 19.

How Does the Brain Actually Work?

Welcome to Brain Function 101. This is a very simplified look into brain function. Let's just start with two main areas of the brain. The first is the *cortex* – that outside covering that looks like a bunch of tubes

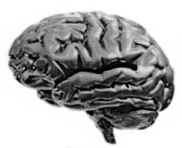

The Cortex

that are connected. It is really quite thin (about 3/8 to ½ inch), but is the hard wiring of basic functions and memory patterns. It is composed of billions of nerve cells called *neurons* which are connected together to form neural patterns. The cortex has a division that is responsible for different yet linked activities. There are areas for speech, specific muscle areas, vocabulary, abstract thinking and much more. The second area of interest is called the *limbic system*. This portion of the brain is one of the oldest in human development. The autonomic nervous system is seated in the limbic portion. The autonomic system controls the critical life support actions such as breathing, heart rate, blood pressure, and many other activities that you do without having the need to be consciously aware. Just imagine what it would be like to have to remember to tell your heart to continue to beat while at the same time breathing, and walking; yet this and thousands of other activities are going on every second of your life without your conscious involvement. This is the job of the autonomic nervous system, which has two divisions - the sympathetic and the parasympathetic. The sympathetic division is responsible for survival when any threat is recognized, while the parasympathetic division is responsible for recovery and healing.

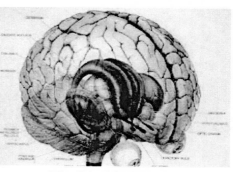

The Limbic System

Our systems have developed a range of ideal responses that include reactions to stressors and what we call normal life activities. These responses directly involve the state of limbic activity. Our memory patterns in the cortex supply information to the limbic system so that any lessons we have learned in the past that affect our survival can be transferred to the limbic system for action. A great example of this is the hot pot lesson. It does not matter how many times you tell a child not to touch the pot because it is hot, the child will have to touch it. The memory, driven by pain receptors, imprints the lesson into cortical memory patterns. This is how we learn and build memories.

Survival is the driving force behind brain activity, but just how the brain works has been the focus of research in neuroscience over the last fifteen years, and what has been revealed is changing the entire health field.

At this point, let's consider the difference between actions such as sleep and awake. These two represent different states of consciousness. Different brain activity determines whether you are asleep or awake. The brain generates what are called brain wave patterns of electrical activity that govern your state of being. Being awake or being asleep is merely a state of brain function.

There are 6 primary brain wave states:

1. Delta brain waves - deep sleep (.5 to 4 hertz)

2. Theta brain waves - light sleep – dream sleep, rapid eye movement (4 to 7.8 hertz)

3. Alpha brain waves - conscious relaxation, meditation state (7.8 to 12 hertz)

4. Sensory Motor Rhythms (SMR) – motor activity and ability to remain clear thinking (12 to 15)

5. Beta brain waves – wide awake, focused, alert (15 to 41 hertz)

6. Gamma brain waves – moments of connectivity, "Ah-Ha" moments, short duration (above 15 hertz)

As the brain moves back and forth through these frequencies, our activities reflect our state of being. If Delta is the primary frequency, we are then in deep sleep, or if in Beta we are in defense and highly aware. The higher the frequency, the more energy is required, thus Beta uses a huge amount of the body's energy. Beta is primarily a defensive survival state and therefore little to no energy is available for healing when you are in Beta.

Healing energy is found at the Alpha, Theta and Delta frequencies. The ability of the brain to move freely back and forth between these frequencies is critical for good healthy body responses. One of the definitions of neuroplasticity is this ability of the brain to shift frequencies with ease as demanded by the body's environment.

At this point, stress enters the picture when it comes to health. If your brain response patterns are not able to adapt quickly and appropriately to the environmental challenges, you have a stressed system and the result is a less than ideal response to stressors. Over time, these add up and the system begins to break down. Remember that closed loop system? When one part of the closed loop malfunctions, it will affect other systems until there is a massive breakdown. This is what happens when your brain loses the ability to adapt ideally (that is, either it is in defense mode or in recovery) and the system becomes unbalanced, or in other words, there is a loss of neuroplasticity[1].

Understanding stress, stressors, and how they exist in our lives is the first step in looking at health, and/or disease[2] in a new way. This is the reason the first part of this book has been dedicated to stress, stressors and to the reason the current medical models of disease control need to be changed.

Some of the new concepts in the approaches to health are already making their way into care programs. The role of stress in challenges such as diabetes, cardiovascular illness, and cancer are becoming more evident.

Chapter 19 - Things To Consider

As the brain is the control system, any level of brain malfunction will affect all the other systems.

If the brain becomes "stuck" in one frequency there are severe consequences.

New information on brain function is changing what we think about the cause of disease.

We need to review the current accepted methods of dealing with illness.

Our learned lessons guide our responses.

Some of those learned responses may be based on incorrect information.

References

1. Does Stress Cause Disease? It Doesn't Help, Reviewers Say - By Neil Osterweil, Senior Associate Editor, MedPage Today Published: October 10, 2007 - Cohen S et al. "Psychological Stress and Disease." JAMA 2007; 298(14): 1685-1687.

2. Stress and Neural Wreckage: Part of the Brain Plasticity Puzzle --- Gregory Kellett has a masters in Cognitive Neurology/Research Psychology from SFSU and is a researcher at UCSF where he currently investigates the psychophysiology of social stress. SharpBrains.com.

###

Recently, I've been especially impressed with the Koren Specific Technique (KST). KST is a low force chiropractic technique that uses instrument adjusting with no popping or twisting of the spine. No x-rays are needed for the KST evaluation since the occipital drop reflex indicates where subluxations (misalignments, fixations, blockages, imbalances) are located. This work is ideal for any age and is very gentle.

This approach addresses the spine and pelvis as well as bones of the skull, face, TMJ, sternum, clavicles and all extremities—shoulders, elbows, wrists, hands, hips, knees, ankles and feet. KST is great for correcting injuries suffered from falls, strains, auto accidents, sports injuries and activities of daily living. It's so gentle that we can adjust cranial bones of babies born with difficult labor, forceps and other stresses to the skull. KST can detect nutritional deficiencies and stressors such as excess chemicals and heavy metals. It can be used to adjust misplaced organs and valves.

Finally, KST can help correct blocked or stuck emotions that may contribute to emotional and physical symptoms. I shared two such cases in the Awareness chapter but here's one more. "Keith", a fifty-year old health nut, had suffered with tightness and discomfort along the left side of his body for several years. Despite trying every natural healing approach he knew, nothing helped. He heard about KST and wondered if it might help. My evaluation showed there were emotional, structural and nutritional causes involved. Small wonder that other approaches hadn't done the trick. The KST emotional assessment revealed the emotion "death" occurring at age four, resulting in tension of the meninges, the fibrous covering of the brain and spinal cord.

I shared this combination of findings with Keith who immediately turned pale. He told me that, at age four, his mother asked him to keep an eye on his two-year-old brother. After awhile, as is normal for a four year old, Keith's attention wavered. Then he heard his brother screaming horribly and saw that he had been run over by the next-door neighbor's lawn tractor. His brother wasn't killed, but he was badly injured and scarred for life.

I adjusted the meningeal tension while Keith visualized the traumatic event. Afterward, I warned that he might experience cathartic dreams or memories. The next visit, he reported: "I cried all evening and had vivid dreams all night." But after that, his left-sided symptoms were much less severe and he was able to release righteous anger toward his mom for putting him in that situation. One year later, he usually has no symptoms and has released the emotional blocks.

Chiropractic definitely is NOT just for back and neck pain and headaches. In the late 19th century, its founder D.D. Palmer, said that disease was caused by structural, chemical (nutritional) and emotional imbalances. KST allows me to evaluate and address all three types of causes.

**(excerpted from Radiant Wellness:
A Holistic Guide for Optimal Body, Mind and Spirit
by Mark Pitstick, MA, DC www.radiant101.com)**

C H A P T E R

T W E N T Y

What are ADD, ADHD, and Autism?

Chapter Twenty

What are ADD, ADHD, and Autism?

Does Stress Play a Factor in These Challenges?

This is a very interesting field of brain research activity. There is some confusion in the public's mind as to the difference between ADHD and ADD - they're both linked together. One is the inability to filter out (what to focus upon - ADHD) and the other is the inability to maintain focus (ADD). ADHD is lacking attention ability or the inability to filter out incoming sensory information and loss of focus. It usually does not include hyperactivity and may even display sluggish and/or spacey characteristics. ADD is about easy distraction (short attention span). They're both attention deficit disorders, so when I use the term ADD, I mean it to include ADHD.

Here is the thing that has been misunderstood about ADD from the start. There was confusion between the hyperactive[1] child and ADD responses in children. The hyperactive child was automatically labeled as ADD because of the amount of activity being mistaken for easy dis-

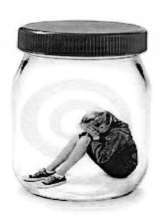

traction. What did not make sense in this labeling was that in taking Ritalin, which is a stimulant, it slowed them down. That doesn't make sense - how does a stimulant slow down a hyperactive person? The people who were classifying the child as ADD couldn't explain this action. New research suggests that stress may affect brain development in children, altering growth of a specific piece of the brain and abilities associated with it.

As we talked with psychologists, we discovered the brain wave patterns for ADD children are way too high in Theta and way too low in Beta[2]. Now, Beta is the wide awake alert response that works on complex problems. It's awake and alert with lots of energy and a true hyperactive child produces too much Beta; it's as if the GO button is switched on all day long. This hyperactive child is not a candidate for a stimulant and, in fact, it can be dangerous. I often wonder about the teenagers who are dropping dead on football fields with heart problems. What is the history? Have they been on Ritalin? Were they on it at the time? When you take someone who is over stimulated and add a stimulant, you put them into a physical stressor that could create a heart attack.

True ADD kids are generating too much Theta and not enough Beta. Theta is subconscious light sleep. When you give them a stimulant that produces Beta activity, they start to react better because their brain is working in a more balanced state. Okay - So what's happening in Theta? Have you ever gone to sleep in the middle of an afternoon and fallen into a super deep sleep? You wake up with a jolt and you can't stand up or figure out where you are? That is the ADD state of too much Theta. The kids in this state are basically sleep walking and the only way for them to function is to keep active. They may take a stimulant such as Ritalin which boosts the Beta production and makes them wide awake and a normal human being for four hours, but only four hours.

How stress plays a role with people who are in high Theta and low Beta.

ADD kids grow up to be ADD adults unless something is done to change the pattern; however, there is more to the ADD story. ADD is a protective measure of the brain[3]. It can be caused from prolonged stress overload or physical brain injuries. With either of these events, the brain goes into chaos; its processing resources are used up and begin to short circuit. If this continues, the individual will experience a complete mental breakdown. We can witness this extreme level of damage with some of the individuals in the street population.

The reason this does not happen to everyone under high stress situations is because the brain has a fail safe program. The innate intelligence within the brain recognizes the danger and shuts off the conscious registering of the stress. Every time there is a stressor, the brain shuts down its Beta responses. The individual just dials out during a stress event and experiences a loss of focus. This dial out may appear as an ADD or an ADHD response. While that helps the individual by not creating more conscious anxiety, the subconscious still has to deal with the increased threat. The subconscious is dealing with the stress information and the message it sends to the limbic system is "danger, danger". The subcon¬scious pushes everything to fight/flight with huge amounts of adrenalin and cortisol being produced. The increase in the stress responses places increased demands on the pancreas and liver as well as on the immune system.

PTSD

We have been made aware of post-traumatic stress disorder (PTSD) because of the wars America has been in for the last ten years. PTSD is a chaotic brain state due to stress overload[4]. The stress can be physical, mental, chemical or any combination of these. We're seeing a lot of people in all walks of life who have suffered from concussions, emotional trauma and/or chemically induced damage. The military used to call this *shell shock*. When people are experiencing PTSD, if you stress them even mildly, such as having them sit in a chair to do a cognitive challenge like a math test, they cannot focus consciously. Their Beta brain activity may drop and their Theta activity may go sky high. When they try to recover after the stressor, they may stay in that aroused mode. The EEG patterns of PTSD are chaotic and the brain activity is unorganized. As they start to heal, the first step is for the brain to develop an ADD pattern.

These brain states place huge demands on the body's systems and cannot be maintained without increased damage. We now know that the primary factor in all aspects of health and illness is our ability to adapt and respond to the stressors in our life. This simple knowledge is the greatest development in the health fields.

Autism

We have an increased incidence of autism in North America and there are many theories as to why this is so. Some blame vaccinations or genetics, and others say no one has an answer. We do know that there are some areas in the brain that are vitally important for autistic responses. The corpus callosum is one area and is responsible for the transferring information from one hemisphere to another hemisphere. The hemispheres need to exchange information. If they don't, people become one sided in their response. If they are right sided, they are much more emotional. If they're left sided, they're much more logical. It happens that most girls tend to be autistic towards the emotive side and most boys tend to be towards the logic side[5],[6]. It is the left brain activity that is the reason why you see the boys in activities such as spinning plates. What they're doing is minutely studying the patterns. They're intrigued by it. Girls tend to become very emotive, liking connection and becoming emotional.

The latest information on autism parallels what we learned about dyslexia. When dyslexia was first discovered, everybody who was dyslexic was super dyslexic. They couldn't read because everything was backwards, or they couldn't do math, and communication was a challenge. As time went on, we realized there were stages of dyslexia. For instance, having a challenge with hyphenated words at the end of a sentence and not being able to put the two parts of the word together is a dyslexic problem. We realize there is a floating scale and dyslexia is not thought to be as disabling as it once was.

In testing as early as 2007 with the Stress Response Evaluation (SRE) provided by the NeuroInfiniti, we were seeing some odd responses such as an inversion of the heart rate (HR) and recovery during the emotion testing (the noises test). Where HR should go up during the stressor and down during recovery, it was reversed. Then we started to notice there were other activities that were abnormal during the noises as well. One of the key factors in looking at autistic patterns is how people respond to noise/emotional tests. Autistic individuals do not respond well to noise. They don't like lots of noise and they extremely withdraw. All of these responses can be seen on the SRE report. These individuals are very sensitive and because there is an emotional factor connected with autism, the social relationship is directly involved. The most important point to be made is that Autism, ADD or dyslexia are all brain function challenges. They are spectral disorders which mean the reactions can cover a wide range or levels (from few to severe) of responses. Therapies that have shown results in the improving of brain function need to be addressed when discussing any of these conditions.

Chapter 20 - Things to Consider

What do you think would happen if you gave an over aroused nervous system a stimulant?

Kids are being diagnosed with ADD just because they are very active.

Stimulants work to activate brain activity but only for a short time period.

The ADD brain wave pattern is a protective fail safe mechanism to prevent circuit breakdown.

PTSD is a brain state of complete overload – ADD is a recovery state.

An autistic brain sees the world differently than does a normal brain.

There are degrees of Autistic responses and aversion to noise is a key sign.

References

1. Difference Between ADD and ADHD By Keath Low, About.com Guide Updated August 02, 2010About.com Health's Disease and Condition content is reviewed by the Medical Review Board - add.about.com › Health › ADD / ADHD › Understanding ADD/ADHD

2. Both Loss of Concentration And The Most Creative Thinking Is With The Theta Brain Wave - Posted on March 16th, 2010 by David in Theta Brain Wave - Brainwave Mind -brainwavemind.com/theta-brain-wave/theta-brain-wave/

3. The Relationship Between PTSD Symptoms and Attention Problems in Children Exposed to the Bosnian War - Syed Arshad Husain - University of Missouri-Columbia-Maureen A. Allwood - University of Missouri-Columbia - Debora J. Bell - University of Missouri-Columbia   Journal of Emotional and Behavioral Disorders

4. Battle Concussions Tied to Stress Disorder By Benedict Carey - Published: January 31, 2008www.nytimes.com/2008/01/31/health/31brain.html

5. What Autistic Girls Are Made Of - By Emily Bazelon - Published: August 5, 2007

6. How autism affects boys & girls differently - By: WMAR Staff http://www.abc2news.com/dpp/news/health/how-autism-affects-boys--girls-differently#ixzz2IAb7A3i2.

CHAPTER
TWENTY-ONE

The Road Less Traveled

Chapter 21.

The Road Less Traveled

The Challenge

It has been a fundamental position of chiropractic that we deal primarily with the nervous system. There was a misconception that arose at the beginning of chiropractic when it was founded by D.D. Palmer in 1895. There wasn't much known about the nervous system and the brain, and little science was available at that time. So the concept of chiropractic came about because of D.D. Palmer working on the spine and bringing back a patient's hearing. It wasn't based on treating a disease or illness. In his words, "I found a bone racked out of place and I racked it back in[1]."

There was a misconception at that point, plus a very poor choice of words used to describe the action. His misconception was that moving bones of the spine, because they were pressing on a nerve, created a hearing change. That has been a theory in chiropractic since that time. Early chiropractic was presented as vertebral misalignment and subsequent nerve root pressure was considered the cause of disease. Chiropractors begin making claims they could cure everything from polio to cancer by moving the bones of the spine. These claims as well as a lack of scientific support for the nerve root *vertebral subluxation theory* has kept the chiropractic profession as a second rate health profession.

In my 32 years of practice I experienced incredible responses from patients under care and quickly realized that there was more going on than simply moving a vertebra. There were times when the responses were the result of a light touch technique or an instrument adjusting technique. The only instruments used to measure changes at that time were x-ray machines. As these x-ray films were static pictures of the bone and joints, they had no connection with the changes in neurological activity that I was seeing. I was at a loss to explain how these events were happening in my own and other chiropractic offices. The introduction story about Kim was the turning point in my life. It started my search to discover how and why chiropractic adjustments could bring about such incredible results.

Every chiropractic educational institute continues to focus on the relationship between the spine, its joints and chiropractic adjusting techniques. The vertebral subluxation[2] is still part of the core belief, but the concept of nerve root pressure is down played as a result of a lack of supportive evidence. Today the colleges have shifted toward the role of joint mechanics and reduction of signs and symptoms. This shift has created a severe restriction in the scope of chiropractic with the result being that events like Kim's or Doug's stories will no longer be seen.

The breakthrough came when I first heard about Electroencephalograph (EEG) work and biofeedback in the early 70s. I met some people doing biofeedback and I was very interested in the fact they were working with brain patterns. I had a feeling that there might be a relationship between chiropractic and biofeedback; however, I never had the opportunity to follow up on this concept until 1993.

In 1993 I met Dr. Annette Long in Colorado and had a new world of possibility opened to me. It was the same time that the 1990s decade of neuroscience research on the brain was underway and the new knowledge of brain function was shaking the scientific world by its roots. Dr. Long and her husband, Dr. Alvah Byers, had been pioneers in the world of bio/neurofeedback. Our friendship led to having many conversations about brain function and at one point in 1999, I suggested that the reason the chiropractic adjustment worked was that it directly altered brain function. My suggestion was not warmly received. Dr. Long suggested that we test my theory. We set up a trial test. Dr. Byers did an EEG. I then did an adjustment. We waited twenty minutes; Dr. Byers did a follow up EEG. We did this on five people. The results showed that there were significant changes. Dr. Byers, being a true researcher said, "Maybe it was just us or the room. It's not enough to make any conclusions."

We started out doing a *null hypothesis*, which is to prove the theory does not work. A "Null Hypothesis" in this case, is a theory based on gathering evidence that the chiropractic adjustment does not affect brain function. We arranged for Drs. Long and Byers to travel to chiropractic events over the following three years, during which we continued to do pre and post adjustment EEG measurements.

The Null hypothesis was quickly discarded due to the incredible alterations we were seeing in EEG studies on post reports. Now we needed to determine what changes were happening and the significance of these changes. We were seeing huge changes in EEG patterns with the chiropractic adjustments, even when using an adjusting instrument or only adjusting one area.

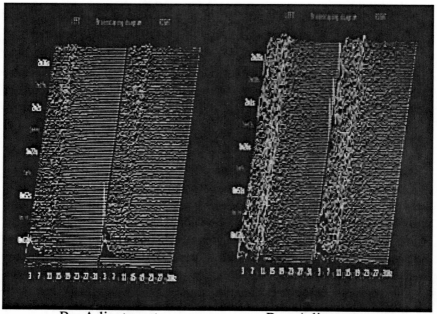

Pre Adjustment   Post Adjustment

These shifts in brain wave activity through a single chiropractic adjustment were so dramatic that according to Dr. Byers, it would take experts in neurofeedback between 50 to 200 sessions of neurofeedback to get that level of alteration. This new view of the power of a chiropractic adjustment to alter brain activity was a shock to all of us and opened the door to the missing link for the chiropractic profession.

When you change brain wave activity, you change how a person relates to their environment. When you change how a person relates to their environment, you change their life. Suddenly it started to make sense as to why chiropractors have seen miracles walk in and out of their offices throughout the years. The basic theory from 1895 of nerve root compression due to vertebral misalignment did not support these miracle responses that have been part of chiropractic history. Since there was no science to support them, they were dismissed as some sort of magic or just a story. The last twenty years of neuroscience research has provided the missing support and knowledge.

I published a paper[3] in 2004 on the work we had done regarding chiropractic and brain function. Today two more papers[4],[5] have been published that support this position.

Now there is a huge movement afoot worldwide. I have spoken to chiropractic colleges, universities, and associations throughout the world and I can see a shift happening within the profession to where we can finally explain the chiropractic "miracles" from a logical, scientific neurological point of view that we never had available before. So it's a very exciting time when we can see that the adjustment actually changes central nervous system function and that's why we got the results over the years. Concepts that govern a profession don't change quickly or easily and the educational institutes are even slower to shift their positions. Strong evidence based research is having its effect and a new understanding of the power of chiropractic care is redirecting the profession. As usual, there will be resistance, and there is a group of philosophically based chiropractors who see the new information as a threat to the theory of vertebral subluxation (bone on nerve) and an attack on the validity of the profession. B.J. Palmer, who is considered to be the developer of the chiropractic profession, said this. "When facts are known, knowledge exists. When we possess knowledge, faith and beliefs disappear, for one is the skeletal frame for substance of the other."[6] The very man whom the philosophical group holds as their mentor and founder of their position supports the development of knowledge that has brought about this change.

Chapter 21 - Things to Consider

Due to limited knowledge, the theory of chiropractic was based on assumptions that no longer can be supported.

When knowledge replaces theory it does not devalue the application of chiropractic.

The updated neuroscience in support of chiropractic increases the role of the adjustment.

Back and/or neck pain are only symptoms of inappropriate neurological function.

Educational institutions are the last bastions of old concepts.

References

1. The Art, Science and Philosophy of Chiropractic, The Chiropractor's Adjuster – D.D. Palmer - 1910 Pub Palmer College

2. "Subluxation is a complex of functional and/or structural and/or pathological articular changes that compromise neural integrity and may influence organ system function and general health." - J Can Chiropr Assoc 2002; 46(4) 215 - EF Owens * Director of Research - Sherman College of Straight Chiropractic

3. The effect of the Chiropractic adjustment on the brain wave pattern as measured by EEG. - Richard Barwell, DC; Annette Long, Ph.D.; Alvah Byers, Ph.D; Craig Schisler, B.A., M.A., DC. International Research and Paper symposium 2004 - Sherman Chiropractic College

4 Cervical spine manipulation alters sensorimotor integration: A somatosensory evoked potential study - Heidi Haavik-Taylor*, Bernadette Murphy -Human Neurophysiology and Rehabilitation Laboratory, Department of Sport and Exercise Science, Tamaki Campus, University of Auckland, Private Bag 92019, 261MorrinRoad, Glen Innes, Auckland, New Zealand Accepted 11 September 2006 - Clinical Neurophysiology 118 (2007) 391–402

5. Cerebral Metabolic Changes in Men After Chiropractic Spinal Manipulation for Neck pain. - Takeshi Ogura, oc, PhD; Manabu Tashiro, MD, phD; Mehedi Masud, MD, phD; Shoichi Watanuki; Katsuhiko Shibuya, us;Keiichiro Yamaguchi, MD, phD; Masatoshi Itoh, MD, phD: Hiroshi Fukuda, MD, phD; Kazuhiko yanai, nro, prro

6. Up From Below the Bottom - B.J. Palmer Vol. XXIII - 2nd edition – 1979 - Sherman College

CHAPTER

TWENTY-TWO

What is the Relationship Between
Chiropractic, the Nervous System and Stress?

What is the Relationship Between Chiropractic, the Nervous System and Stress?

Your signs and symptoms indicate that your state of health is less than ideal; you have a bad neurological pattern or abnormal neurological responses. While these patterns may have been appropriate at a given

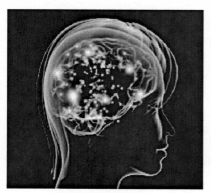

moment, your system is now unable to recover. For instance, the constant stress in your life has created the fight/flight response in which your brain waves tend to stay mostly in Beta. You are no longer able to really relax. Your sleep pattern is disrupted. The limbic part of your brain gets the message to stay in defense. This pushes the autonomic nervous system to the sympathetic

side, so up goes your heart rate and blood pressure. The problem with this motivation is that there are situations where the neurological response, while appropriate for a short term situation, becomes fixed as a long term pattern. Your nervous system gets stuck in that pattern because you've been under constant low grade stress so much that the sympathetics are consistently elevated. This becomes established as your "normal" neurological pattern. The greatest example of this lies in the fact that cardiovascular challenges (CVD) are the number one cause of death in North America[1]. This includes high blood pressure and heart distress up to and including irregular heart rhythms and physical damage, all of which occur as a result of stress levels causing the system to remain in high alert for a long period of time.

What does the Chiropractic Adjustment actually do?

Here is what we have recently discovered about the chiropractic adjustment. What we thought we were doing, that is, correcting vertebral misalignments to reduce pressure on the spinal nerve roots, is not the case. Current research has shown that the chiropractic adjustment is an extremely effective neurological pattern interrupt. The adjustment creates a barrage of sensory information directly into the central nervous system. This sensory input creates a change in the nervous system[2]. Anytime you can get the nervous system's attention to a point where it's starting to react, it means you have an opportunity to change the negative pattern back to a more balanced pattern. This alone is the foundation for the effectiveness of chiropractic from the very start and supports why all of the various techniques in chiropractic get results.

This research has completely altered the chiropractic profession and is not unlike discovering that the world isn't flat. There are still many out there who have a challenge with a regard to change when new information comes along; however, the impact of this new understanding widens the potential and range of chiropractic care.

The chiropractic adjustment allows the brain to break the patterns. It allows it to reset itself to a more positive ideal balance. This understanding of the role in neurological pattern interrupt also explains the application of acupuncture, massage therapy, Rolfing and many other forms of therapies used today. In fact, it includes the effects of drugs. They too create a pattern interrupt in order to be effective, but in so doing create other system imbalance challenges known as side-effects[3]. They are not side effects. They are direct effects, just conveniently misnamed so as not to reflect the danger in use.

Duration of Care

There have been other studies that have been going on for years in other fields regarding the effectiveness of pattern interrupt, such as neuro-linguistics.

The brain views *survival value* as its primary goal[4]; it will always move toward a better neurological balance direction. The innate or inborn

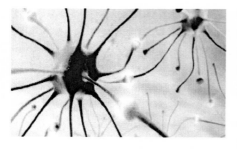 intelligence in the body wants to maintain a proper balance and given any chance, it will try to reset itself to a more appropriate pattern.

The second goal deals with the benefits of ongoing care. Chiropractors are well known for telling patients that they need ongoing care. This has always been a challenge because of the selling overtone when chiropractors recommend lifetime type care, especially when the pain complaint has been corrected. As we now look past symptom relief toward improved neurological function, long term care plans not only make sense but are neurologically justified. The adjustment program is about neurological retraining which takes time and repetition[5].

Many times medical practitioners are challenged by the duration of chiropractic care programs and the reason is that they have no concept of the neurological retraining done by the adjustment. Remember that the medical profession is "signs and symptoms" removal based. As chiropractic is based on a process of retraining, just like training for any physical activity, the method of care is different from the typical medical model. In the medical model you may visit the doctor two or three times over the course of care; however, you are involved in medical care daily with the prescriptions provided. Chiropractic is a contact profession and by that I mean many office visits over the course of the care program. The reason is that the care is directed to retraining your nervous system. This takes repetition and time. Here is an example.

Try this easy exercise. Take a few seconds and sign your autograph. You've been signing it for many years. How long is it going to take you to sign your autograph just as well with the opposite hand as you can with your normal hand? It's going to take a long time to do that. Where is the information stored that allows you to sign your autograph? Between 95 and 98 percent is stored in the brain with the balance in the muscles of the forearm and hand. What happens if you only practice once? It's never going to get any better. You have to build new neurological pathways, new dendrite (nerve cell) connections and new neurons that connect with one another in order to sign well with the other hand. To make it work correctly, you have to do it repeatedly, over and over and 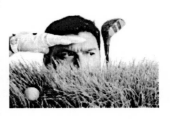 over again. Repetition is the key way to change neurological patterns. This is the reason for the longer care programs that are recommended by most chiropractors. Any golfer knows the value of repetitive training to groove their swing. If you don't train your swing well - the photo tells the story.

There are many Chiropractors today who are only interested in pain relief and offer short term care recommendations. This type of care works well to relieve symptoms, but does little to address the long term neurological challenge or cause of the problem.

If you want to deal with the cause, you must have pattern interrupt re-training. There are several ways we can do pattern interrupts to overcome the cause of your challenges. We have found that one of the most dramatic and effective methods of altering a neurological pattern without any side effects is the chiropractic adjustment because it doesn't have the negative effects of drugs, surgery or electroshock therapy.

You may wonder why every stimulation does not reset the neurological pattern, if all it takes is a pattern interrupt. The answer is to be found in the word *appropriate*. The application of either an appropriate or ideal stimulation needs to be considered in order to have the best effect[6]. If the established pattern is one of over-arousal of the nervous system, then an appropriate application should be one that quiets down the nervous system. If the pattern is under-aroused, then the stimulation should be to speed up the system.

Chapter 22 - Things to Consider

- Does this change your understanding of chiropractic care?

- Can you see how the concepts of chiropractors being, "back doctors" or "back crackers" diminishes the role of chiropractic?

- Since stress directly involves the nervous system, as does the chiropractic adjustment, can you see that there is a direct relationship between the two.

- While most patients who visit chiropractors have some form of health challenge, because of the past concept of spinal involvement, most have no idea that chiropractic has a much broader role in maintaining health.

- Old explanations of chiropractic application, such as postural studies, pain reduction or putting joints "in" that are "out" no longer apply.

- Chiropractic is based on a neurological retraining process, not a chemical substitute.

- Chiropractic does not deal with drugs or surgery
  .
- Bad brain patterns are the cause of all health challenges and those patterns can be changed.

References

1. CVD causes more deaths in the USA than the next 5 leading causes of death combined (National Health and Nutrition Examination Survey III, 1988-94)

2. Enabling Function and Well-Being Dunn W. Implementing neuroscience principles to support habilitation and recovery. In: Christiansen C, Baum C, eds. Occupational Therapy:. 2nd ed. Thorofare, NJ: SLACK Incorporated; 1997; 186-232.

3. The Epidemic of Overmedication - By Siri Carpenter - http://krist.newsvine.com/_news/2008/11/17/2121091-the-epidemic-of-overmedication

4. The Anatomy Of Fear and How It Relates To Survival Skills Training - By Darren Laur - www.lwcbooks.com/articles/anatomy.html

5. Myths About Stroke Recovery - Posted by admin on November 30, 2010 - strokerehabonline.com/tag/neurological-rehabilitation

6. Brain Economics: - Housekeeping Routines in the Brain - Proefschrift ter verkrijging van het doctoraat in de Medische Wetenschappen aan de Rijksuniversiteit Groningen op gezag van de Rector Magnificus, dr. F. Zwarts, in het openbaar te verdedigen op maandag 5 oktober 2009 om 14.45 uur door Paolo Toffanin geboren op 12 maart 1979 te Sandrigo, Itali"e Promotores : Prof. dr. A. Johnson Prof. dr. R. de Jong Prof. dr. G.J. ter Horst Copromotor : Dr. S. Martens Beoordelingscommissie : Prof. dr. M. Eimer Prof. dr. B. Hommel Prof. dr. N.M. Maurits ISBN (boek): 978-90-367-3979-5 ISBN (digitaal): 978-90-367-3978-8

###

Jonah's Story

Jonah is a nine year old boy referred to us by his mom's co-worker whose daughter had a great reduction in bedwetting and behavioral improvement under chiropractic care at our clinic. His parents were desperate to improve his behavior as it was dramatically affecting his school performance and destroying their family dynamic. After many years of drug and psychotherapy, his behavior continued to progressively worsen and he became more disconnected.

At his first visit we conducted a consultation and stress response evaluation and it showed dramatic under-arousal of his brain and exhausted nervous system. My stress response specialist who performed the scan reported that as she brought the patient to the scan room and set him up he never made eye contact or conversed. He simply followed her and nodded to answer simple questions. His hands were damp and cool and he could not sit still.

Jonah's parents then watched as I performed his first KST adjustment. Immediately his constant movement and nervous tics quieted. He took a really deep breath and flashed a rare smile. His very skeptical dad brushed off a tear, turned and walked to the front desk to make an appointment for himself. I cautioned the parents that although we had a dramatic result that day, retraining the brain is a process and would be a bumpy ride. We scheduled his next visit in 12 days since I was leaving the next day for a weeklong conference.

I held my breath waiting for the family at Jonah's next visit and expected them to report only temporary improvement. His mom stated that after leaving the office after the first appointment that they went out to dinner for the first time as a family since Jonah was 3 and had a great time. He uncharacteristically spoke to his big sister all the way home and remained happy for several days. Both parents are now chiropractic patients as well and later told me that they thought originally I may have overstated how dire Jonah's stress response test was until they saw that the results of theirs were markedly better and they felt that they were "a mess".

Two short months later his fog has lifted, he smiles and talks constantly and is excelling at school. His mood swings and outbursts have subsided. Neurologically based chiropractic has healed this family and unleashed the potential of a bright and happy boy that now has a reconnected and balanced brain.

Jonah's Continuing Story...

It has now been 6 months since Jonah came under Neurologically Based Chiropractic care. As his brain balance continues to improve, his affect and performance also improve along with his family life and socialization. Prior to starting care he was combatant and nearly non-communicative. At his visit yesterday, he was engaging a room full of people, confidently and happily showing off his skill in completing an intricate puzzle that most people (including me!) cannot figure out. He initiates conversation, jokes and flirts with girls in the clinic. After his adjustment I told his Mom that I wanted to update colleagues on his case and asked what changes she could report and she replied tearfully "you have no idea what you've done…you have no idea". She composed herself and in a stream of consciousness quickly composed the following list of what first came to mind: calmer, able to receive feedback, talks to many people (previously mom or dad ONLY), able to make tough decisions and understand consequences, can sit for extended periods of time without "meltdown" (can eat out and shop again), communicates needs and wants, no longer aggressive when angry and he "graduated" from behavior therapy last week!

In about a month Jonah has a fresh start in the fifth grade. His new teacher is excited to work with him (a first) and now that his potential has been unleashed he's starting on par, and above grade level in math. The sky is the limit because Dr. Richard Barwell and his incredible team developed and foster the paradigm of Neurologically Based Chiropractic and train us to apply it through the NeuroInfiniti. This equipment accurately assesses brain function in many children like Jonah and when this assessment is combined with a masterful chiropractic technique like KST, created by Dr. Tedd Koren, the synergy elegantly enables Doctors of Chiropractic to effectively correct what's found on the stress response evaluation. I am humbled and blessed to stand on the shoulders of these brilliant Chiropractic visionaries. We all, patients and doctors alike, must help them tell the story and further the dream, saving countless millions of children like Jonah.

Patrick J. Keiran, DC
Keiran Chiropractic, PA at Paradigm Wellness
259 Main St.
Jay, ME 04239
www.KeiranChiro.com

TWENTY-THREE

Instruments that Deal with Stress Responses

Chapter 23.
Instruments that Deal with Stress Responses

Computers have changed the face of health care today. Research methods are much more accurate and we now have the ability to see brain activity as it happens. Instruments such as functional MRI or PET scans have revealed more about how the brain functions than we could have even imagined twenty years ago. Many of these instruments are extremely expensive and take many years of training to be able to use. The development of an instrument called the Electroencephalograph or EEG has brought very valuable information on brain function into the field of neuroscience at a much lower cost factor.

When the EEG was first developed in the1920s, it was without the capabilities of a computer, so all of the interpretation had to be done manually. Today computers are capable of running the entire testing and interpretation within minutes. This has made the EEG usable and affordable in office use. EEG scans are very reproducible and accurate[1].

The value of EEG studies with their direct relationship to health has been well established over the years by the fantastic work done by psychologists. Thousands of studies and research papers have established the viability of not only the accuracy and reproducibility of EEG but also the role cortical function plays in brain function[2].

As usual, however, anything new or outside current medical thinking always brings challenges, and the acceptance of EEG work has been no exception. Today EEG is well established as a clinical and research tool for understanding brain function. Working with two pioneers in the field of EEG and neurofeedback, I experienced the value of watching cortical ac-

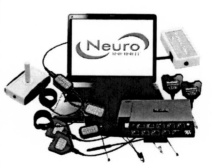

tivity in action live time. This brought me to a company called Thought Technology, based in Montreal, Canada, with whom I worked to develop an instrument called the NeuroInfiniti™ (NI).

The NeuroInfiniti

We now have certified methods of stress response measurement; a test called the Stress Response Evaluation or SRE. The Neuro-Infiniti now offers the ability to present printed reports on cortical activity (via EEG) as well as six different neurophysiological responses to both stressors and recovery. It is now possible to see the state of dynamic brain activity without using expensive equipment such as MRI or PET scanners. The NI can show abnormal cortical activity and the effect it has on the other base systems of the body, before signs and symptoms appear. Heart Rate Variability

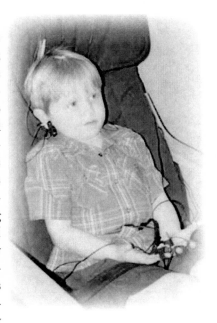

(HRV), which is included in the analysis program and was developed by the cardiologists of America and Europe[3], represents the application of this new approach. HRV has the ability to reveal damaging heart activity even before the abnormal blood chemistry shows up.

We devised a system with the NI of doing a dynamic analysis of central nervous system function that measures what is going on in the cortex (chapter 19) and how it influences the function of the limbic system. The limbic system is the seat of the autonomic nervous system (chapter 19) which includes both sympathetic and parasympathetic activities. In other words, we can see how people adapt to and recover from different types of stressors in their lives. It also allows a look at the neurological patterns that have been established as compared to ideal patterns.

We use a baseline of eyes open and eyes closed. Next the NeuroInfiniti uses a cognitive (ability to think) challenge (the dreaded math test) and then recovery. There is an emotional challenge (important noises) and then recovery and then a physical challenge (a simple breathing exercise) for three minutes and then recovery. This provides us with a dynamic test with which we're able to look at cortical function, heart rate, heart rate variability, hand temperature, skin temperature, respiration rates and shoulder tension or general muscle tension from stress recovery in the body.

This test is completed in a short twenty minute examination which allows us to see how the nervous system handles different types of stressors and how it recovers from them. In administering the SRE, the NeuroInfiniti instrument doesn't care whether you're a medical doctor, a dentist, a chiropractor, a para-professional, a massage therapist, a dietician or a professional assistant. The NeuroInfiniti simply tells us about the state of central nervous system function as com¬pared to ideal responses. The NI represents a huge advancement into the emotional driven neurological responses that have become our stress response patterns and therefore the way we control our health challenges.

One of the other instruments we found to be of great value is through a company called PorterVision and is called MindFit.[4]

MindFit Neuro-Trainer®

We started looking at how we can access the central nervous system to be even more effective without any side effects.

We tested the MindFit (formerly ZenFrames) by using live time EEG recordings during the 20 minute sessions. We saw in the patterns with the EEG that the MindFit absolutely shifted the brain wave patterns on people and it had them experience brain wave patterns that were hard to achieve in the conscious state. The patients experienced what it was like to get true relaxation or true focus. When the brain loses its ability to operate in an ideal frequency, the brain loses its neuroplasticity (its ability to adapt to its environment), which means it reduces its survival value.

The retinal (back of the eye) flashing and the binaural sound (alternating sound to both ears) of the Mind Fit. is like opening a doorway of possibility for the brain. The brain loves it - it says this is what I've been missing and the flashing lights and alternating sounds gives the brain an opportunity to experience a new stimulation. An example is one in which a person's Theta frequencies (light sleep, subconscious state) are not working correctly which is really an ideal state for healing and health promotion, so they have not been experiencing good sleep patterns. They're disrupted through the day. This person cannot properly relax. They have too much Beta brain activity and are burning up too much energy.

When we suggest they need to dial in more Theta, they don't even know what we're talking about. It's beyond them consciously. Trying to explain the Theta sensation is rather like explaining chocolate cake. If you've never had a piece of chocolate cake before, and you ask me what it tastes like, my answer is going to be, "Well, it's kind of rich, it's kind of earthy and it's sweet and - it is an experience -you have to taste it." It's the same thing that happens with the MindFit. People get to experience what Theta actually feels like. The brain gets to dial it back in again and the brain knows. Once it tastes it, once it understands what it feels like, it's much easier for it to return there. So the MindFit is invaluable in this whole series of bringing people back to a healthy state. The MindFit experience is called brain wave entrainment.

What Comes Next

The point is that today we not only understand that our health challenges are not caused by some outside factor but that it is our body's systems which are malfunctioning and impairing our ability to adapt and respond ideally. The latest research now has established that this malfunction is totally controlled by the Central Nervous System (CNS)[5] and that is where the primary challenge to our maintaining great health lies. We are all becoming aware of the failure of medication to address the cause of the problems in that it is designed to treat symptoms only and now the danger of over-medication is killing thousands of people each year.

As we work toward the close of this book and offer information about how you can change your health picture, please, keep in mind that your loss of health took time to develop and it will take time and commitment from you to rebuild. The instruments discussed offer, first of all, a picture of the challenges to your neurological function (the NI Stress Response Evaluation {SRE}) and second, methods for you to retrain your brain function to more appropriate patterns.

Chapter 23 - Things to Consider

- Computers have changed our understanding of health functions.

- The development of EEG instrumentation has allowed us to see the cortex of the brain in action and established our different states of being. (Being awake, being asleep, being relaxed).

- There is now instrumentation that can record your states of neurological response and recovery as compared to ideal.

- These states of response and recovery can be retrained to more appropriate patterns.

- These retraining programs do not involve drugs or surgery!

- The instruments mentioned deal directly with the cause of the challenge, not just the symptoms.

References

1. For the EEG, the sensitivity was 86.4 %   - Reproducibility and sensitivity of detecting brain activity by simultaneous electroencephalography and near-infrared spectroscopy -   Experimental Brain Research -October 2012, Volume 222, Issue 3, pp 255-264 -Martin Biallas, Ivo Trajkovic, Daniel Haensse, Valentine Marcar, Martin Wolf

2. The electroencephalogram (EEG) is a measure of brain waves. It is a readily available test that provides evidence of how the brain functions over time. - Electroencephalography (EEG) -Author:Diamond Vrocher III, MD Coauthor:Mark J. Lowell, MD Editor:William C. Shiel Jr., MD, FACP, FACR

3. Heart rate variability refers to the regulation of the sinoatrial node the natural pacemaker of the heart by the sympathetic and parasympathetic branches of the autonomic nervous system.   The Expert Series interviewed Dr. Robert Nolan. www.behavioural-medicine.com/articles/hrv/001.html

4. Eliminate stress, reduce pain, stop smoking, and even lose weight with the help of the PorterVision. Creative Visualization Relaxation Device - www.portervision.com

5. Current medical research states that 95% of all diseases/illnesses are cause by stress. Comprehensive Stress Management, by Jerrold S. Greenberg, 1990

CHAPTER
TWENTY-FOUR

What does a neurological stress test tell you?
What is heart rate variability? (HRV)

What Does a Neurological Stress Test Tell You?

As you have been working your way through this book, I hope that by now you have been able to look at health and illness from a new perspective. This new perspective hopefully includes how vitally important it is to look to the root cause of our loss of health; whether it be infections or body system failures. All illness has as its root cause our loss of ability to adapt to stressors[1]. The nervous system is the primary controlling factor in our ability to adapt. The NeuroInfiniti instrument was designed to test the nervous system's ability to react to four major types of stress that we all experience in life, and then its ability to recover from them. The test offers information about cortical function and limbic system responses. The efforts in the previous chapters have been directed at offering a clearer understanding of why you get sick. The remaining portion of this book is directed at how you can regain control of your health challenges. While some of the neurological responses you may be familiar with, such as increased heart rate or high blood pressure, others may be new to you and some explanation is needed.

What is Heart Rate Variability? (HRV)

Heart rate variability was developed by cardiologists in America and Europe[2]. Heart rate variability is the difference of your heart speed when you breathe in versus when you breathe out. Your heart rate speeds up when you breathe in and should slow down when you breathe out. In slowing down the heart, it gets a chance to rest, recover and heal. If your stress level has unbalanced your HRV, the heart does not slow down; it just keeps going at a steady beat so that it never gets a chance to rest and relax. A person can have a normal heart rate (pulse) and still have very poor heart rate variability. They are separate heart functions. If poor heart rate variability continues, you will end up with heart damage. What is the primary killer in the world today? It is cardiovascular disease, which is why we need to be looking at both the heart rate and the heart rate variability to determine heart health.

We can measure both of those to see how stress affects the heart rate variability and/or heart rate. We've seen young people 21 years old with heart rates of 120 beats a minute when they're just sitting in a chair. We've seen people with low heart rates who have bad heart rate variability with heart damage. We've seen other people with high heart rates and bad heart rate variability including damage who are candidates for a cardiac event. Cardiologists developed heart rate variability testing which is a wonderful insight into the workings of the heart and through which we can catch a lot of challenges before they become catastrophic in nature. So heart rate variability is another very important test for neurological health.

The Role of Your Muscles Under Stress?

People are aware that muscles tighten when you're under stress. You always want people to rub your shoulders. That's because the muscles that run from your shoulders up to your neck to support your head, are the first ones to tighten under stress. The primary muscle involved in this action is called the *"trapezius"* and is the only muscle with a unique nerve supply. Its nerve supply comes directly from the brain. The brain recognizes that it is sitting at the top of this flexible column that can get damaged, and when damaged severely cause death. It acts like a turtle and tucks the head down. When those muscles tighten up they literally reinforce the neck so you don't get a broken neck. When that happens it restricts the motion in the neck and causes all sorts of problems. One of the signs of long term stress is the flattening of the ideal cervical (neck) spinal curve.

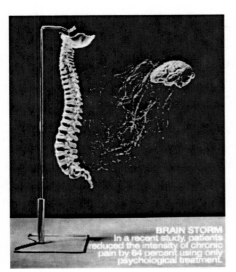

BRAIN STORM
In a recent study, patients reduced the intensity of chronic pain by 64 percent using only psychological treatment.

This protection is not just with the big muscles. It's also the muscles of the jaw and face. The brain knows - you have a jaw that's important in staying alive because it chews food to keep you going. If you get hit in the face, the jaw may break, so your brain clenches your jaw during stress. Keep tightening the facial muscles and you end up with migraine headaches or TMJ problems. The low back pain that chiropractic is so good at relieving is created by muscle spasms due to a stress response. Your low back problem is really a brain function problem![3] If the stress has upset the nervous system so badly that you're now showing signs in the big muscles and the muscles are going into spasm, what is it doing to the muscles that make the gut work or any of the other body functions?

The Role of Stress in Digestion?

Stress does the same thing to these muscles. They tighten up. You go into survival mode and at the moment of figuratively running away from the bear continually, digestion is not important so it stops. Then you get putrefaction in the gut. Now you've got digestive problems. You're not going to start getting proper nutrition out of your food because it's not breaking down properly. We see a lot of people with these problems. The digestive process breakdown also tends to store fat, and it gets stored around the belly. That's what happens under chronic stress.

In America, not only do we have not only bad nutrition habits but also the stress levels are so high we're seeing a huge amount of obesity. There are people walking around with huge bellies, most of it because of stress that's out of control in their lives. All the focus on gluten free foods is just because of the relationship between stress, the immune system and digestion. The body has become sensitized to gluten, which then shuts down the digestive process. Dropping gluten from your diet does not address the real cause of the problem. The real problem lies within the central nervous system malfunction[4].

Along with the above, remember that under stress hand temperature drops because the blood gets pooled away, the skin conduciveness increases, heart rate increases, heart rate variability starts to fall apart, muscles get tense, respiration goes up and becomes erratic. These are all factors that we can measure as to how you're doing in your life with stress and your ability to recover.

Warning signs: Type 2 Diabetes: is it a stress problem?

With all this muscle tightening, heart rates going up, high stress loads, high energy demand, fight/flight responses, along with consusing a enormous amount of fatty foods, we are creating massive demands on the body's systems to keep up. The brain consumes about 30 percent of the body's total energy, which is the most energy of any system in the body. That energy has to come from somewhere. You have to take your food and digest it; it is broken down so the body can use it. That is the job of the liver and pancreas, to make the digested food into usable food for us, which is directly related to how the pancreas functions[5].

Stressors place a high demand for energy production. This energy comes from the food we eat which involves the organs responsible for in braking down that food into usable energy forms. The liver and pancreas play vital role in this energy production.

Compare this to a car running at 150 miles an hour that was designed to run at 90 miles an hour. There are going to be some breakdowns. The high energy demand puts such huge stress on the pancreas and the liver that it can't maintain. Remember, the liver is a filter. It takes out the toxins in the system. If you start to interfere with liver function, the toxins are not getting removed as they should. The nervous system still has to deal with this and puts even more demands on the pancreas. Finally the pancreas burns itself out and can't do it anymore. When that happens we're now into diabetes. Just before it completely burns out, the body shows signs of type 2 diabetes, a warning sign telling you that the pancreas is overstressed. It's in trouble and if you don't do something about it, it's going to crash and burn. Luckily you can change your diet, get regular exercise to help the body stay in balance, and get some control over what's going on in your central nervous system.

Other responses that are signs of stress patterns

Cold hands. Your hands become cold because the blood is shunted away from the extremities and brought into the big muscles so that you can use them to fight or run. As blood is the prime factor in heat regulation, the loss of blood in the extremities drops the temperature. Chronically cold hands are a sign of a chronic stress response. The ideal temperature range for hands is 94 to 97 degrees F or 34 to 36 degrees C.[6] Your hand temperature should go down during stress and warm during recovery.

Skin conductance (SC) or galvanic skin resistance (GSR). The skin needs moisture to stay healthy; however, there is an ideal range of moisture which is .8 to1.5µS (µS is the unit of measurement used for Skin Conductance). The hand moisture increases during a stress response so that your grip improves. In fight situations, this would be a good thing. If this response is continually on alert, the system will shut down and your hands will then become very dry. This would show as very low, below .5 skin conductance.[7] Ideally your SC should increase during stress and drop during recovery.

Respiration. Breathing rates should increase during a stressor and decrease during recovery. Ideal respiration rates vary between 6 to12 breaths a minute.[8,9] Breathing rates should go up during stress and down during recovery. The one except is that during a relaxing breathing exercise, the breath rate should go down.

All of these responses should vary during stress challenges and recover during relaxation. They increase during stress and drop during recovery with the exception of hand temperature which works the opposite.

Chapter 24 - Things to Consider

- Has this information offered a new understanding as to why we get sick?

- Does the concept of your role in your health challenges give you hope to change the patterns?

- Have you ever wondered why your hands were cold all the time or your blood pressure high?

- Does it make more sense to change your response patterns than to start taking drugs to cover up the symptom?

- Does all of this information just make it easier to take a pill for short term relief than to want to work at changing your neurological patterns?

- Smoking, poor diet, lack of exercise, poor relationships, work stress, lack of rewards, electromagnetic exposure, money challenges, drugs (legal and illegal) ultraviolet exposure, and other life challenges go on every day. They are accumulative in nature. Has this information caused you to stop and look at your life?

References

1. Current medical research states that 95% of all diseases/illnesses are cause by stress. Comprehensive Stress Management, by Jerrold S. Greenberg, 1990

2. Heart rate variability standards of measurement, physiological interpretation, and clinical use. Task Force of the European Society of Cardiology and the North American Society of Pacing and Electrophysiology. Circulation 1996; 93:1043-65.

3. Brain Study Of Back Pain Sufferers Yields Intriguing Results; Scans Show Amplified Pain Signals In Patients With Back Pain Of Unknown Origin Science News Oct. 28, 2002 — ANN ARBOR, MI

4. Celiac Disease (CD) is a lifelong inherited autoimmune condition www.celiac.org/index.php?option=com_content&view...id...

5. Personality correlates of adherence to type 2 diabetes regimens. Hyphantis T, Kaltsouda A, Triantafillidis J, Platis O, Karadagi S, Christou K, Mantas C, Argyropoulos A, Mavreas V: Int J Psychiatry Med 2005, 35:103-107. PubMed Abstract | Publisher Full Text

6. Information on Extremity temperatures - Clinical Science Journal, Psychophysiology Journal, Headache Journal, Biofeedback and Self-Regulation Journal, The American Journal of Clinical Hypnosis, Proceedings of the Biofeedback Society of America, Journal of Clinical Psychology, Behavior Therapy Journal, Journal of Consulting and Clinical Psychology, American Journal of Psychophysiology, British Journal of Psychiatry, etc

7. Essentials of Anatomy & Physiology. ^ Martini, Frederic; Bartholomew, Edwin (2003). San Francisco: Benjamin Cummings. p. 267. ISBN 0-13-061567-6.

8. Control of breathing. In: Physiology, Castro M. Berne RM, Levy MN (eds), 4-th edition, Mosby, St. Louis, 1998.

9. The regulation of normal breathing, Douglas CG, Haldane JS, Journal of Physiology 1909; 38: p. 420–440.

CHAPTER
TWENTY-FIVE

How Your Brain Can Fix It!

Who's in control?

Chapter 25.

How Your Brain Can Fix It!

Who is in control?

The most exciting aspect of these new concepts is that you are the one who is in control! You don't need to look outside yourself for the cause of your health challenges. The problem we have is that we live in a world where we have been carefully taught that the only way to good health lies with drug therapy. This teaching includes the belief that all we have to do is get some drug prescribed and everything will be fine. When you add the power of the media behind those medicine ads, your brain starts to imprint the message. Media's ability to alter our perception is very subtle yet very dangerous[1]. Whether you see it or hear it, the message is accessing your thought processes. This is the reason television is the main portal for pharmaceutical ads. They imprint through both sight and sound plus portray a strong emotional image in the process. Then they repeat the message over and over. Our perception is that public media must always tell the truth so everything advertised must be safe. The media has created how we think about our health and how we heal. Sorry folks, but you have been had, and it is time to do something about it. We are finally discovering that the message is not always necessarily true. The government has finally made the drug companies start putting the truth on television by listing all the side-effects, even though they distract you with nice graphics while listing all the nasty effects. Have you noticed that a lot of the side-effect symptoms look like what the drug was designed to alleviate in the first place, plus more? What happens when you start using chemicals in the body is that it may have a favorable response for that specific symptom, but it stresses the body in other areas because the drug puts the system out of balance. It makes other things worse.

The answer to good health is not to be found in introducing another stressor by way of a drug. The answer is that first we need to recognize that the cause of the problem lies in abnormal neurological function and then seek ways to address the cause directly. The question needs to be, "What can I do to get my nervous system back in balance?" The interesting thing about all of this is that it is very easy to do. You can be taught how to warm your hands in a very short period of time. You can just sit there and learn how to neutralize the effect of cold hands. People say to me, "Well, my hands are always cold, that is normal for me.". No, that's not normal. It just tells you that your nervous system has been damaged to that point where it's not able to run normally.

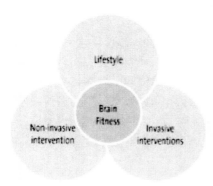

You can be taught how to remedy that very quickly by using some brain techniques that are at the forefront of the modern world of health. Once you learn that, once you learn how to warm your hands by how you think, you will realize that you're the one who created the cold hands in the first place. The power of this ability to alter your neurophysiological functions just by how you think will give you back control of your life. Since you are the one who created your health challenge, you are the one who can fix it!

Where to start

We know that the chiropractic adjustment is extremely effective as a neurological pattern changer, which is what it was intended to be from the beginning of chiropractic. (Remember, our primary focus has always been the nervous system).

As the research in neuroscience continues to reveal how the brain functions and malfunctions, along with the consequences of the malfunction, it has become evident that the reason for the success of chiropractic over the years deals directly with its ability to alter brain function. Chiropractic detractors have always been more than willing to dismiss any claims of positive results as placebo, anecdotal (stories), or just plain fraudulent. Even with the latest research that supports everything in this book, the detractors will not change. Change is difficult, especially when the communication media bombards the population with information that states drugs are the answer to everything. The school system is based on the medical model even though the latest information and research says differently, so real change will take time. The change process must be able to withstand all out attacks. This is the way it is! It is now up to you to govern your actions based on what you have read and whether or not it makes sense to you to put the information you have learned to the test.

Find a chiropractor who has read this book or is a neurologically based practitioner. Even better, find one who is using instruments such as the NeuroInfiniti and/or MindFit. Don't expect to stay for only one or two visits. Remember that in order to change neurological patterns, it will take time, repetition and training. The seriousness of your health challenge, the duration of the complaint, and your ability to respond, are all factors at play in your recovery. Some care plans may be once a week for six months or a year, just to move your system back to a level of stabilization. Other plans may be three or more times a week for four to fifteen weeks. It all depends on your specific neurological needs.

Many chiropractors will not tell you these types of plans as they are afraid that you won't even start care. Just remember that the back pain that seems to have just started yesterday has actually has taken years to develop and just yesterday that little movement you did was really the straw that broke the camel's back (pardon the pun). With this in mind, starting with the most powerful non-invasive form of care that will start the process of changing your neurological pattern makes good sense. Get chiropractic care!

The next step is fun and intriguing. It involves the world of *bio-feedback* and *neurofeedback*. This field has also come under the scorn of the medical profession as it is also outside of the medical model of care. The primary intent of these forms of care involves the retraining of neurological patterns by self-driven reward programs. Basically you play various types of games on a computer or instrument that rewards you when you achieve a specific goal.

Any programs that involve limbic system activities such as respiration, heart rate, hand temperature, skin conductance or muscle action are called biofeedback. Any activity that directly involves cortical brain wave patterns is called neurofeedback. Both are extremely effective in helping you build new neural patterns which can replace those old patterns that are causing your health loss.

When you combine chiropractic and the feedback training, you are using very powerful tools to change your life.

Before we go one step further, I need to make something very clear - neither chiropractic nor either feedback program treats you for any disease. The treatment of disease is the practice of medicine. Chiropractic and feedback are not medical treatments. What they are lies within the concepts of functional neurology. That is, if the nervous system is working ideally, then you have the ability for good health. The loss of good health is not the result of too little Tylenol in your system, but in damaged neurological function, to the point of causing signs and symptoms as a warning. The goal of care needs to be how we can return your ideal neurological function without any side effects.

Today we can lay out a course of care that's much more appropriate for each patient. Further and importantly, we can make sense of our care to others in the healing professions because all of a sudden we're talking a language they can understand with a neurological foundation.

Knowledge has the power to change the world in which we live. Knowledge has lengthened our life span and reduced the level of sickness and disease. It has provided us with increased comfort and free time. Knowledge continues to create the opportunity to change and grow but is not always welcomed. This holds true within the health professions and yet we now stand on the greatest breakthrough in the knowledge of the cause of disease in the history of mankind. Many unanswered questions of the past, including the great mystery of spontaneous remission of serious diseases can now be explained and understood; however, it requires letting go of concepts such as the germ theory on the part of medicine or the nerve root compression theory in chiropractic.

This book challenges some old theories but only because of our increased knowledge in brain function and its role in maintaining a healthy balance between healing and defense. This new information exposes our need for an ongoing search into neuroscience and its relationship to health. There are times when new knowledge makes a previous theory incorrect and times when it just opens the door for a better working model. This book involves both of those aspects. Traditional approaches are deeply imprinted and any suggestion that there is another way will be challenged and trashed before any consideration is given to the material. Look at the history of the introduction of new concepts and one would wonder why anyone would be willing to propose a new idea.

My life has been a dedication to my profession and I have been rewarded. One single Kim or Doug experience is reward enough. There were many more similar experiences and each one far beyond the current public perception of the role of chiropractic. These cases may have presented at my office with back pain, but as we worked through their care, they began to recognize that other health challenges were disappearing. Chiropractic care response takes time and repetition because we are retraining neurological patterns. To the patients reading this book I say, "Look to your nervous system for the cause of your health challenges and for your recovery. Stand in awe at the design of how our systems work and recognize that the power lies within you to change your world. Take back control of your life!"

The message of the book is not only a call to health professionals to stop and consider the power of this new information in their practices, but it is also to the public, so that they can recognize that they too play a major role in the gathering of new knowledge to guide their health actions.

Chapter 25 - Things to Consider

- You are the arsonist and the firefighter in your life.

- The power of the media including print, TV, radio and THE INTERNET affects how you think.

- If you created your neural patterns then you can change them.

- When you change your patterns, you change how you respond to your environment.

- When you change how you respond, you change your life.

- When you can control how you respond to stress and improve your ability to recover, you reduce the effects of stress; you reduce the inflammatory process and restore health.

- Chiropractic adjustments alter nervous system patterns.

- It took time to build your neurological patterns; it will take time and training to create new ones.

Reading this book has already started the process of building new patterns.

Now take action!

Start hugging people on the right side (heart to heart).

Take up Yoga and learn to breathe correctly.

Wear your watch on the other arm.

Undo your reaction buttons.

Get Chiropractic care!

Start Bio and/or neurofeedback.

Buy the MindFit and use it everyday.

Start walking everyday.

See your MD to get off meds – not to take more.

Have a glass of Red wine and some dark Chocolate every night.

Get seven hours of sleep each night.

Listen to relaxing music.

Reference

1. The Shallows – What the Internet is doing to our brains - Nicholas Carr - W.W. Norton Publisher ISBN 978-0- 393-33975 -8

BONUS-CHAPTER

TWENTY-SIX

High-Tech Solutions for High-Tech Stress
by Patrick K. Porter, Ph.D.

Chapter 26.

High-Tech Solutions for High-Tech Stress

By Patrick K. Porter, Ph.D.

In the middle of a scorching summer heat wave in 1987, I attended a convention in Las Vegas, Nevada. It was only a few months after the opening of our new enterprise in Phoenix, and I really couldn't afford to be there. My curiosity got the better of me, however, when I discovered that new mind technology would be introduced at that event.

I was rushing to my next workshop when a female voice called out to me. I glanced at the woman who smiled at me as she stood in front of her booth. I waved and smiled at her. "I don't have time," I said. "I'm late for my next workshop."

Then a strange electronic device perched on the table behind her caught my eye. I touched the machine. "What's this?"

The woman stroked the device as if it were her beloved pet. "*This* is the Sensory Input Learning System. We call it SILS for short," she said. "I'm Linnea Reid." She shook my hand then signaled to a middle-aged man sitting beside the machine. "This is my partner, Larry Gillen," she added.

"Would you like to go for a ride?" Linnea asked.

One of my early loves was electronics, so I couldn't resist giving it a try. "Sure," I replied.

Linnea told me to lie back in a reclining chair. She tucked a blanket around me and handed me a set of earphones and a pair of sunglasses equipped with small LED lights. "I'll let you go about ten minutes," she said. "Just close your eyes and have a great trip."

Not knowing what to expect, I settled into the chair and closed my eyes. Within moments my senses were awakened by the rhythm of flashing lights and tones. An immediate feeling of relaxation and well-being washed over me. Now this was something I could get into.

By the time the session ended, I was blown away. I had never before felt so relaxed. I didn't want to move. "Come on," Linnea said as she shook me, "the group is about to take a break. You need to get up."

"That was the most amazing ten minutes of my life," I said.

"Ten minutes? That was more like forty-five minutes. You seemed to be having such a good time, I decided to let you keep going."

"Wow! It seemed to go that fast," I said, snapping my fingers. "I've got to have one of these machines. How do I buy one?"

"Well, you're in luck, I happen to sell these things… and the show special is only ten-thousand dollars."

My heart sank. I was a new business owner. She might as well have said ten million dollars. Yet I had never let money stand in my way before. I simply had to own one of these amazing devices. The wheels in my mind began to turn.

As fate would have it, Linnea and Larry relocated to Mesa, Arizona, and opened their business, Light & Sound Research, a short distance from my clinic. I attended several of their demonstrations and we soon formed a friendship.

One night, we sat in a diner discussing all the possibilities the SILS system offered. "I've got an idea," I said, "what if I sponsor your demonstrations at my clinic and, between events, you can leave the machine with me so I can research the benefits with my clients?"

"I have to admit, I'm pretty tired of hustling around to different locations," Larry said to Linnea. "Sounds like a great idea to me."

"I agree," she said. "Getting some feedback from real clients would be invaluable."

In that instant I once again had accomplished a goal without it costing me a dime. By setting no limitations on how I would possess the machine, I had visualized and realized my goal.

That was 1987. Since then almost every one of my clients, along with the clients who attended programs in my franchise system, experienced this life changing technology. To say the results were astounding would be an understatement.

How is technology changing the way we use our brain?

Light and sound technology, also known as *visual/auditory entrainment*, is introduced to the brain through the ears and optic nerve using computerized technology emitted through headphones and specially designed glasses equipped with light-emitting diodes (LEDs). The lights flash at predetermined frequencies and are coupled with *binaural beats*, which are heard at a low level through the headphones. The visual/auditory entrainment is typically synchronized, but can be varied depending on the desired effect.

The flickering light patterns and binaural beats reach the brain by way of the optic nerve and inner ear respectively. Within minutes the brain begins to match the frequencies of the light pulses and sound beats. The method by which this entrainment occurs is known as frequency following response. Unlike biofeedback, where the user attempts to consciously change brainwave activity, light and sound induced entrainment influences the brain without any conscious effort.

The frequency following response simulates the relaxed brainwave frequencies know as alpha and theta. This is the state in which the individual relaxes and the mind develops focus. Listeners experience a reduction in inner chatter and improved concentration. Because frequency following response is a learned response, the effect is cumulative. After a few weeks of regular use, users gain a sense of balance and inner calm. Most people report feeling serene, focused, and alert even when faced with high-pressure situations. Furthermore, most users report experiencing enhanced creativity and feeling more rested with less sleep.

While light and sound technology can be beneficial to most people, it is not for everyone. Persons with epilepsy, any type of seizure disorder, or any visual photosensitivity are advised against using a light and sound device. People who have a pacemaker, suffer from a heart disorder, have a history of serious head trauma, or are taking stimulants, tranquilizers, or psychotropic medications, including alcohol or drugs, should consult their physician before use. Anyone experiencing dizziness, migraine, or severe anxiety after using light and sound should discontinue using the device and consult a physician.

How do tones create relaxation?

In 1839, an associate professor at the University of Berlin, H. W. Dove, discovered what he termed binaural beats. His early research showed that putting a given frequency in one ear and a different tone in the other causes a person to hear a third tone, which is the difference in frequency of the two tones.

He found that the human ability to hear binaural beats appeared to be the result of evolutionary adaptation and that our brains detect and follow binaural beats because of the structure of the brain itself.

Until a 1973 article by Gerald Oster[8], however, binaural beats were considered no more than a scientific curiosity. Oster's paper was groundbreaking not so much in presenting new laboratory findings, but rather in bringing fresh insight to the topic by identifying and connecting a variety of relevant research performed after Dove's discovery. Oster is credited with uncovering just what effect binaural beats could have on the mind and body. He viewed binaural beats as a tool

How Binaural Beats Work

1. The binaural beat is generated from two separate tones of a slightly different pitch
2. One tone is presented to the left ear and the other to the right ear
3. Your brain combines the two tones to make a single new tone
4. The single tone pulses to match relaxed brainwave frequencie
5. Your brain follows the pattern and creates the relaxed state

for cognitive and neurological research. Moreover, he identified the auditory system's propensity for selective attention (sometimes referred to as the cocktail party effect), which is our ability to tune out distractions and focus on a single activity. Oster also found that Parkinson's sufferers and those with auditory impairments generally could not hear binaural beats. Thus, he concluded that binaural beats could be used for diagnosing certain disorders. He also discovered gender differences in the perception of beats and felt that how a woman perceived the tones could be used to gauge fluctuations of estrogen (the latter assertion rising from a study he replicated that corroborated findings of gender differences in the perception of beats).9

Oster's publication of "Auditory Beats in the Brain," along with his assertion that binaural beats could be created even when one of the frequencies is below the human volume threshold (which supported his hypothesis that binaural beats involved different neural pathways from those involved in our direct conscious perception), launched a wave of new research into frequency following response.

How does light create relaxation?

Almost since the time humans discovered fire, it's been observed that flickering light can cause alterations in consciousness and even inexplicable visual hallucinations. Throughout history, stories abound of tribal elders, healers, and shamans using this knowledge to enhance their practices.

Early scientists, also captivated by this phenomenon, explored its practical applications. Around 200 AD, Ptolemy experimented with a spinning spoked wheel placed between an observer and the sun. The flickering of the sunlight through the spokes of the spinning wheel caused patterns and colors to appear before the eyes of the observer. Many of these observers described a feeling of euphoria after exposure to the light patterns.

Joseph Plateau, a Belgian scientist, used the flickering of light through a strobe wheel to study the diagnostic significance of the *flicker fusion phenomenon*. As he caused the light flickers to come faster and faster, he found that at a certain point the flickers seemed to "fuse" into a steady, unflickering light pattern. In 1829, Plateau dubbed this phenomenon *persistence of vision*. He noted that healthy people were able to see separate flashes of light at much higher flicker speeds than were sick people. Today Plateau is recognized as the first animator. Modern filmmakers still rely on persistence of vision to trick our brains into believing that what we are viewing is actually moving and not just a series of still images.

At the turn of the century, French physician Pierre Janet noticed that when patients at the Salpetriere Hospital in Paris were exposed to flickering lights, they experienced reductions in hysteria and increases

Four Brainwave Frequencies

Brainwave Frequency	Name
13–40 Hz Active thought and concentration; associated with busyness and anxious thinking	**Beta waves** (Reactionary Mind)
7–13 Hz Relaxation (while awake), daydreaming; associated with creativity	**Alpha waves** (Intuitive Mind)
4–7 Hz The place between asleep and awake; associated with deep meditation and sleep learning	**Theta waves** (Inventive Mind)
< 4 Hz Deep dreamless sleep	**Delta waves** (Rejuvenating Mind)

in relaxation.

By 1990, scientists were able to measure the effect of light on serotonin and endorphin levels. In one such study, eleven patients had peridural (the outermost of the three membranes covering the brain and spinal cord) and blood analysis performed before and after participation in relaxation sessions using flash emitting goggles. An average increase of beta-endorphin levels of twenty-five percent and serotonin levels of twenty-one percent were registered. The beta-endorphin levels are comparable to those obtained by cranial electrical stimulation (CES). The researchers concluded that photic stimulation has great potential for decreasing depression-related symptoms.(10)

Why use light and sound together?

While research has proven that both light (flickering) and sound (binaural beats) can produce relaxed states, at Light & Sound Research we found that combining the two could move the body into a more profound level of relaxation; it is the highly kinesthetic state of tranquility that is optimum for healing and accelerated learning.

When I met Linnea and Larry, it was at the dawn of the computer revolution. Microchip technology was in its infancy, and computer engineers were a rare commodity. Nevertheless, Larry and Linnea found an engineer who could program a computer chip to do the work that the therapist previously had to do. With the help of thousands of documented sessions using a *mind mirror* (EEG machine), they discovered which programs worked to optimize the frequency following response and bring about optimum states of relaxation and learning. They then designed the first portable relaxation system and called it the MC^2.

In the next two decades, the franchise company I founded used this light and sound technology combined with SMT to help hundreds of thousands of people facilitate life changes such as losing weight, kicking a smoking habit, or conquering an alcohol or drug addiction. Others used it to eliminate pain, have stress-free childbirth, get motivated, achieve goals, enhance sports performance, improve at sales, and other life enhancements. One gentleman found that that the light/sound/SMT combination ended a five-year battle with chronic hiccups. Another young man came to me with a habitual nose click that even surgery hadn't cured. It stopped during his first session and never came back.

What is the secret to getting these kinds of results?

One of my favorite songs is *Change Your Mind* by Sister Hazel. One of the lines in the song goes, *"If you want to be somebody else, if you're tired of fighting battles with yourself . . . change your mind . . ."* I love this song because I believe the best way, and sometimes the only way, to make changes in your life is to first change your mind. Because images, beliefs, and values are so deeply rooted in consciousness, changes must happen at the other-than-conscious level before they can manifest in your life. In my experience, the light/sound/SMT combination is the quickest and easiest way to change your mind.

If you plant a seed, and know that you are watering and caring for it, you can pretty much sit back, relax, and let it sprout. You wouldn't keep digging up the dirt to see if the seed sprouted, would you? If you did uncover the seed to see if it is sprouting, you would probably stop its growth. I believe that this is what happens when people try to make changes at the conscious level; they set a goal, but then find themselves digging up old images, beliefs, and thought patterns, and end up stopping their growth.

When you relax with light, sound, and SMT guiding your conscious mind, you are free to liberate your other-than-conscious mind. Psychologists would say that you are bypassing the critical factor and letting the other-than-conscious mind take over. In other words, you plant the seeds of change, then sit back, relax, and let them sprout.

What are the Best Light & Sound Parameters?

A good choice for a frequency following response program that produces deep relaxation starts at a state of high cortical arousal, a beta frequency of say 15 or 16 Hz. It then ramps down by gradually changing frequency until reaching slow alpha (8 Hz). The frequency should stay there for about seven minutes of the session and then ramp up to a moderate, relaxed alpha (10 Hz). Some programs ramp down into the theta range (4 -7 Hz) in order to achieve a deep other-than-conscious experience. Light and sound combined with positive suggestion, creative visualization, deep relaxation, soothing music, nature sounds, or a combination of these, creates heightened states of awareness.

While there is a wide assortment of relaxation training systems—

autogenic (self-produced) training, progressive relaxation, meditation, and biofeedback to name a few—most of these take conscious effort. With the breakthrough of light and sound technology, you don't have to "believe in" or "do" anything. Through the frequency following response, the brain "syncs" to the strobe light and binaural sounds. You are in the experience and don't have to create it.

As an example, if you and I were to go to a secluded beach on a beautiful day while the sunlight reflects off the water and the waves rhythmically pound the sand, and if, while in this environment, we discussed the life improvements you would like to make, chances are good you would enjoy the conversation and accept any advice I might offer. Because of the environment created by this seaside walk, we would be synching to an alpha state, or about ten cycles per second.

Now if we were to have this same conversation on a bustling street in downtown Manhattan with horns blowing, lights flashing, vendors yelling, and rapid footsteps all around us, we would be synching to high Beta, or about eighteen cycles per second. The results would be very different. During the city walk, you might get distracted, frustrated, or nervous. In this state, you would be much less open to a conversation about improving your life, and would probably reject any advice I may give, even if it's logical advice. Are you starting to see why brainwaves are so important to our well-being?

What is the Benefit in Achieving the Alpha and Theta States?

As you learned about the fight-or-flight response and into the relaxation response is the best step you can take to overcome the brutal effects of stress. The relaxation response can't happen as long as you generate high beta brainwave activity. Your brainwave activity must dip into alpha, which I refer to as the "intuitive mind," or theta, which I call the "inventive mind."

Because theta is the threshold of sleep, it is best known for lucid dreaming. A person in this state often cannot separate thoughts about his or her awakened state from the lucid dream state. Many believe that theta is the optimum state for creativity and that it's the only place one can make a quantum leap in consciousness. Unfortunately, the theta state is difficult to maintain. When you slip into theta (4-7 Hz), which everyone does at least twice each day (right before falling asleep and just before awakening), and when there are no beta or alpha frequencies mixed with the theta, most people lose consciousness. This is where the frequency following response comes in—it keeps your brain engaged. When people use a light and sound device, they often describe feeling as if their inner experience is more real than the outer experience, which is temporarily suspended.

Researchers might say that these people have entered stage-one sleep, sometimes called the twilight state or the *hypnogogic* (from the Greek *hypnos*, meaning sleep, and *agnogeus* meaning conductor) state. While this is a very healing state, and one that heightens the visualization experience, it was not often used for the purpose of teaching relaxation skills. I believe the results achieved by the thousands of clients who have used the light/sound/SMT combination in our franchise programs proves that when a person sees, hears, and experiences the life changes they desire in the alpha and theta states, those changes come to pass in the physical world more quickly and with far less effort.

What are the Benefits of Light and Sound Technology?

Whenever people ask me why I'm so passionate about light and sound technology, I tell them one of my favorite jokes. It goes something like this: One evening a man in a tuxedo rushed up to a street musician and asked, "How do you get to Carnegie Hall?" Without skipping a beat the musician answered, "Practice, man, practice!"

SMT works because it involves mental practice or *spaced repetition*. In my opinion, there is no faster or easier method for achieving spaced repetition than through the synchronized rhythm of light and sound. The induction into higher brainwave states increases brain activity, while the induction of lower brainwave states reduces hyperactivity and feelings of anxiety. Brainwave entrainment within alpha states, for example, creates relaxation and a decreased stress response by providing a slower and more relaxed brainwave state. A faster brainwave state, produced by faster flickering of the LED lights, induces a higher brainwave state, and is theorized to enhance brain stimulation and increase cognitive abilities. In many cases, a faster brainwave state can decrease hyperactivity, similar to the paradoxical application of neurostimulant medications such as Ritalin and Dexedrine.

Research showing the efficacy of light and sound technology is not uncommon. Creative visualization (SMT) and stimulation of brain wave activity are among the most studied areas of psychiatry and psychology. The following results have been demonstrated through numerous studies and in my own experience with thousands of clients:

- Increased long- and short-term memory
- Increased attention span and concentration
- Reduction of anxiety and depression
- Reduction of medication intake
- Increase in right-left visual-spatial integration
- Major increase in creativity idea generation
- Easier decision making and holistic problem solving
- Decrease in migraine or headache frequency and intensity
- Reduction in PMS and menopause symptoms
- Reduction in insomnia and sleep disorders
- Improvement of motivation

"The only way to discover the limits of the possible is to go beyond them into the impossible."

Arthur C. Clarke

BONUS-CHAPTER
TWENTY-SEVEN

Unlocking Your Health
At The Speed of Thought
by Patrick K. Porter, Ph.D.

Chapter 27.

Unlocking Your Health At The Speed of Thought

By Patrick K. Porter, Ph.D.

Achieving your life and health goals can be as easy as taking a breath in open air. The trick is in learning how to use your mind to get what you want.

Whether you realize it or not, at every moment you are affirming something for your life. When it comes to your body, you are either affirming health or you are affirming illness. Which tells us that healing starts with a thought.

An American Indian elder once described his own internal struggles this way: "Inside of me there are two dogs. One of the dogs is mean and evil. The other dog is good. The mean dog fights the good dog all the time." When asked which dog wins, he reflected for a moment and replied, "The one I feed the most."

We use this elder's story as a metaphor about how our minds work. When you give thoughts energy, or when you feed them with emotion, they will grow. This is true whether the thought is good or bad, harmful or helpful. The purpose of this chapter is to teach you how to feed the right dog—the healthy dog. Using positive affirmations does all this.

What is a Self-Mastery Affirmation?

An affirmation is a specific statement that elicits a response. Affirmations can be either spoken or written. For maximum benefit, they should always be stated in the positive. Affirmative declarations, when stated consistently, help you visualize and realize your goals. By affirming what you want each day, you are doing something positive toward fulfilling your dream of losing weight and keeping it off.

It has been said that a picture is worth a thousand words. If this is so, how does a spoken or written word change your self-image?

Well, that's where Self-Mastery Affirmations come in. We train you to use specific language patterns that create the mental pictures you want. By using positive affirmations, you are the producer and director of your inner theater; you are directing your mind to create what you want. In other words, you become the "Steven Spielberg" of your mind!

People tend to use a great deal of thought power on what they don't want instead of what they do want. Unfortunately, your mind tends to give you exactly what you dwell on, which, in this instance, is what you don't want.

As an example, imagine that you are a business owner and have just hired a new assistant. You spend the entire first morning training your new assistant on everything you don't want her to do. When you are finished, you leave for lunch.

What is your assistant going to do?

You guessed it, everything you don't want her to do. After all, what choice does she have when you never told her what you want? Another answer may be: Nothing at all. Again, she doesn't know what to do!

I once counseled a middle-aged man named Tony who desperately wanted to beat his buddies on the golf course. The only problem was, no matter how hard he practiced, his game seemed to stay the same or worsen. He sat in the chair across from me and frowned. "I practice and practice but nothing happens."

This was the opening I was looking for. "What did you just say," I asked.

"I practice and practice and nothing happens," Tony repeated.

"Then you're getting exactly what you ask for," I said.

Tony stared at me with unblinking eyes. "What do you mean," he asked. "That's not what I want."

"I know," I said, "that's why you're here. Unfortunately, you've been practicing affirmations without the proper training."

Tony's eyebrows shot up.

"The way you speak to yourself has powerful implications," I said. "That's why Henry Ford said, 'Whether you think you can or think you can't, you are right!' The same is true with your golf game. Whether you think you will improve or not improve, you are right. What would you prefer happen with your golf game?" I took out an index card and handed it to Tony. "I mean if your wildest dreams could come true?"

"I would break ninety consistently," he answered.

"So, would an affirmation like, I am scoring at an 89 or lower,

make sense?"

"Yes, I think that would work." Tony replied.

"Then go ahead and write it down in your own words. Just make sure it's stated in the positive."

After Tony had written his affirmation, I asked him to place the card in his pocket. "Whenever you notice an unwanted thought about your golf swing," I said, "just stop yourself and then take out the index card and read it. Better yet, when you hear the inner negative thought, say to yourself, backspace/delete, and then take out the card and read it. Read it out load whenever possible."

Tony looked pensive for moment. He then touched the pocket with the affirmation card tucked inside and smiled.

"See," I said, "it's working already." His smile broadened.

"This is only one piece of the puzzle," I reminded him, "and it takes practice. Your mind operates through your senses and they all play a roll."

For Tony this was significant in relation to his golf game, but he also found that the habit of affirming his goals and desires had a positive effect in many other aspects of his life.

So what about you? What words do you regularly say to yourself in regard to your body or weight? What pictures do these words create in your mind? What emotions arise? Let's take a moment to determine what kind of self-talk you have going that might be limiting your ability to lose weight.

Do you have any of these negative affirmations scripting your life?

If you can answer yes to any of the following statements, Self-Mastery Affirmations are your key to re-scripting your life.

1. Do you make negative statements or have negative beliefs about yourself that you repeat internally throughout the day?

2. Do you use negative statements about yourself in your every day conversations with family, friends or coworkers?

3. Do self-deprecating remarks negatively influence your behavior, such as causing you to procrastinate?

4. Do you still believe the negative comments made by members of your family or friends when you were young?

5. Do you replay negative feedback you get from your spouse, boss, teacher, colleagues, children, parents, and relatives? Does this get in the way of achieving your goals?

6. Do you have a negative self-image of any part of your body that you visualize, and then allow it to influence how you present yourself to others?

7. Do you have negative self-talk based on assessments others have made of your competency, skills, ability, knowledge, intelligence, creativity, or common sense?

8. 8. Do you have negative stories about your past behavior, failures, or performances that you systematically run through your mind and that influence your current conduct?

9. 9. Do you have a negative attitude about your potential for

achievement? Does this attitude influence your motivation, stop your effort, and kill your drive?

10. 10. Do you have feelings of guilt, either real or imagined, that prevent positive inner thoughts?

11. 11. Do you discuss negative prophecies that you or others have made about your future, your success, your relationships, your family, or your health; do these haunt you as you face a daily struggle to "win" at weight loss or at the game of life?

12. 12. Do you use negative visualization or self-talk to your personal detriment?

How do you change these internal messages?

Your best thinking brought you to this very moment. If you aren't getting what you want, then you will need to upgrade your thinking. Unfortunately, you can't go to the corner software store and purchase the latest upgrade. But don't worry; we'll work together through Self-Mastery Technology to turn you into your own software engineer for your mind.

The first step in programming is to know the language you are using; in our case, we'll be using the language of the mind.

What we say and what the mind hears can be completely different. For instance, let's imagine we are at a family function and little Jimmy is running toward the door. Someone yells, "Don't slam the door!" Jimmy runs out and...SLAM! The next thing you know poor Jimmy is sitting in the corner in time out. Jimmy has no idea why he's being punished. In his mind, he did exactly what he was told to do. You see, the subconscious mind doesn't know how to process a negative. When Jimmy heard, "Don't slam the door," his mind created a picture of him slamming the door.

Here's a great example. If I ask you not to think about dancing pink elephants, what happens?

You can't help but think about them, right?

To be a software engineer for the mind is to eliminate negative thoughts and replace them with statements that are affirming. This seems simple enough on the surface, but putting it into practice is another matter. This is where the Self-Mastery Technology comes in. A good engineer will have a proto-type, which is a working model, but not a production model. If the proto-type works, it will then go into production.

The affirmations you will create here should be thought of as proto-types; if they work in the laboratory of your mind, you will then put them into production in your life.

Now here are Some Tips for Writing Self-Mastery Affirmations

Always state what you want in the first person (I or I am). State your affirmation in the positive and as if it is occurring or has already occurred.

Examples:

"I am living a slim lifestyle one day at a time."

"I am enjoying my body at 145 lbs or less."

"I am drinking health-giving water daily."

"I am a healthy person."

"I am excited to be at my ideal weight."   ...and so forth.

Now give your affirmation energy. Empower it with emotion.

Imagine yourself fulfilling the affirmation. See it in full living color, hear the sounds, and imagine how you feel while living the affirmation. In other words, engage all your senses.

Let's use the following affirmation: "I look great at parties and easily say no to Candida-causing foods."

When you read the affirmation, are you picturing your shoulders rolled back? Is your head high?

What are other factors that would convince you that the affirmation is true for you? What are you hearing? What happens when your favorite music is in the background? There are no limits in the imagination, so feel free to dream up precisely the life you want. Be sure to write all affirmations in your own handwriting. Read the affirmations aloud, with emotion, at least once a day so you can be reminded of their intrinsic value.

Most people have spent the greater part of their lives telling themselves what not to do and we all know that doesn't work! Your mind is starving for the loving tone of your own voice reinforcing positive thoughts and patterns.

In my book, Awaken the Genius, Mind Technology for the 21st Century, I have a section about affirmations and how they work. We go deeper into this area by discussing what I describe in my book as impact words.

So Just What is an Impact Word?

An impact word is a word or series of words that has a direct impact on you. As an example, if learning were important to you in the context of your job, you would be drawn toward employment ads that use the term learning in its description. As an example: Seeking intelligent, resourceful person to help develop weight-loss programs. Must be willing to learn and apply new knowledge to help clients get noticeable results.

Impact words also house our values or trigger our value system when they are used. These words help run meta-programs, or the programs of the subconscious.

How can these words be of benefit to you?

First, if you know what these words are, you can use them to create more powerful affirmations and more beneficial behaviors. Continuing with the example of learning, if you use that word in you're Self-Mastery Affirmation, it will have more impact. Example: "I enjoy learning and applying information about a healthy lifestyle."

Second, you can find out how these words are giving energy to unwanted behaviors. Let's use the example of the word, challenge, which is a somewhat common impact word. Many of the clients I see will tell me they enjoy a good challenge. If they are having trouble losing weight and "challenge" is one of their impact words, the excitement of the "challenge" inherent in losing, or not losing, weight may be working against them, and may override the benefits of being naturally thin. The person might even have a negative response to the word 'thin," because they feel they were passed by when the "thin" genes were handed out. They can look at a thin person and get angry without knowing why. In this case, desire for a challenge and the goal of being thin are in conflict and the person will not lose weight. To correct this habit, an effective affirmation might be, "I enjoy the challenge of thinking and eating like a healthy person."

Now let's discover your impact words so you can get started putting them to work for you.

At the top of a blank sheet of paper write down the word "Job." What has to be present in a job for you to enjoy it? Write down the answers that come into your mind. Some past clients gave answers like:

1. a challenge

2. freedom to do it my way

3. flexible hours

4. a stimulating environment

5. working with people

6. variety in what I'm doing

Next write down the word "Relationship." What has to be present in a relationship for you to enjoy it? Examples I have heard in the past are:

1. There has to be communication

2. Closeness or a physical attraction

3. Common purpose or goals

4. The person has to be fun loving

5. He or she has to be intelligent

6. The person must be into a healthy lifestyle

Next write down a "Hobby" that you enjoy. What is present in that hobby that causes you to enjoy it? Clients have responded with statements like:

1. Its a distraction

2. Its a challenge

3. Its fun

4. Its stimulating

5. It gets me out of the house

6. It's a creative outlet

Next write down how you know that you have done a good job? You have two choices here. You know when someone else tells you. As an example, Frank just finishes painting the living room. He is unsure if he has done a good job. Then the moment of truth. His wife walks in. She is thrilled with the job Frank did. She comments on how good it looks. At that moment Frank knows the job is right. He feels it inside. He knows when something external, someone else or something else, tells him.

Let's imagine that George paints his living room. He is sure it's done well. He cleans up the brushes and puts away the paint. His wife comes in. She notices a few flaws in the job George did. George then spends several hours convincing his wife that he intended to do the painting that way. George knows he has done a good job internally.

In the area of self-help, having an internal convincer is best because this person is usually internally motivated as well. It should be noted, however, that even the most internal people I know still enjoy a hearty pat on the back for a job well done from time to time.

Now all you need are the four simple steps for putting your impact words into Self-Mastery Affirmations.

Step 1: Let's look at creating a Self-Mastery Affirmation to take action. Using the list of words you wrote earlier, let's imagine you want to start an exercise program. You would add the impact words that motivate you into the affirmation, which empowers the mind to take action. In other words, the meta-program that runs the challenge program or the freedom program now works for your new outcome of exercising.

Sample affirmations would be:

- "I am enjoying the challenge of exercising daily." The impact words her are enjoying and challenge.

- "I am free to exercise in a way I enjoy daily." The impact words are free and enjoy.

- "I am flexible with the exercise I do daily." The impact word is flexible.

- "I am enjoying stimulating my muscles and building a fat burning machine." Here, the impact word is stimulating.

- "I am enjoying a variety of workout routines." The impact word is variety.

Step 2: When you are creating a Self-Mastery Affirmation

about yourself, your self-image, or imagining yourself in a future event, you would impact this affirmation with the relationship words. Let's use the example of learning about weight-loss using the words discovered before.

Sample SELF-MASTERY Affirmations would be:

- "I am easily communicating health information read, heard, and experienced." The impact word is communicating.

- "I am allowing a closeness with new health information and I am physically drawn to learning about ways to get healthier."

The impact words are closeness and physically.

- "I have a perfect recall of information. It is stored in a way that it will serve the common purpose and help me accomplish my goals." The impact words are common purpose.

- "I am experiencing a genuine fun loving attitude about learning how to lose weight and keep it off." Here, the impact word is fun loving.

- "I am accepting my natural intelligence to learn how to take my weight off and keep it off." You guessed it, the impact word is intelligence.

- "I am totally enjoying a healthy lifestyle and am open to learning more." The impact word for this affirmation is healthy lifestyle.

Step 3: Let's take a look at how your hobby-related impact words might help you. Think about it for a minute, how resourceful would you feel if you approached your problems as if they were your hobbies? Well, if you were like my brother-in law, you would spend all your extra time, energy, and money on it. Let me explain . . .

One crisp fall morning, while the world was still engulfed in darkness, my wife Cynthia and I slept on my sisters pull out bed in her living room. We had been forewarned that the boys would be up early to go hunting. Not being hunters, we were completely unprepared for what we witnessed upon awakening.

First, my sister's husband, Russ, walked by dressed in camouflage from head to toe. He had the Rambo look down pat, right down to the bowie knife clipped to his belt. Then came Mikey. He too was in camouflage with a smaller version of the bowie knife at his side.

"Paul, let's go!" Russ yelled from the back door.

Paul, who was seven years old at the time, burst from his bedroom in full hunter garb. He ran through the room, hooking his child-sized bowie knife to his belt.

That afternoon, the fearless hunters returned empty handed.

My wife and I observed this same ritual for three straight mornings, and each day they returned with nothing. My curiosity grew stronger each day. "Russ, what do you get out of this exercise?" I asked.

I love the time with the boys," he said. "And being in nature? There's nothing else like it. Out there, I have time to think . . . and dream. It's just a great break from the daily grind."

Once Russ explained his hobby, it made perfect sense. Before that, I simply couldn't fathom his fascination with getting up at five am to go sit in the cold Michigan woods. But then again, it wasn't my hobby.

I enjoy golfing. I may even be a little obsessed with it—which is true for most golfers. Russ, on the other hand, tells me it is a game for fools. "How else could you get someone to pay $100 to run around a cow field chasing a little white ball? He says.

I spent a great deal of time explaining the intricacies of golf to him. I detailed the reasons I loved the game. I described the excitement of the challenge. I spoke passionately of how the game required a certain level of intelligence to choose the right club, and to know how to swing for every ball position.

"Give me a rifle anytime," was his reply.

At first his answer frustrated me. How could he not understand the thrill in golf? But then I remembered, it wasn't his hobby.

Think about your hobby. How much time, energy, and money have you spent on it this year? What would happen if you put that same kind of motivation into changing something about yourself?

For this exercise, let's focus on your goal to lose weight. Sample

suggestions would be:

- "I am enjoying my healthy eating distraction." Can you guess the impact words here? That's right, enjoying and distraction.

- "I am enjoying my challenge of weighing 145 or less." How about here? If you said challenge, you are correct.

- "I am having more fun eating healthy than I thought possible." Did you recognize fun as the impact word here?

- "I am stimulating my metabolic rate by drinking 8-10 glasses of water." This one might be a little tricky. If you guessed stimulating, you are correct.

- "I am experimenting with a healthy lifestyle that is getting me out of the house." Do you remember this one? The impact words here involve getting out of the house.

- "I am allowing a creative solution to my weight problem of the past." Of course, the impact word here is creative.

Step 4: Now it is time to apply the knowledge of your convincer. Remember, this relates to the question, "How do you know if you've done a good job." If someone or something outside of you must tell you, then your convincer is external. If you know inside, then your convincer is internal.

The other-than-conscious mind works best when you start with the end in mind. What we know about the convincer is that it will work even quicker and easier if we pace your belief about the outcome.

Let's imagine that you want to exercise more regularly. An example Self-Mastery Affirmation for the externally convinced would be:

- "I am enjoying the praise from my friends and family as I exercise 4 times a week."

- An internally convinced sample would be:

- "I am enjoying the quiet confidence I feel after an exercise session."

Do you see the difference? The secret to using the hobby impact word list is using it directly in your Self-Mastery Affirmations. They key is in taking the time to imagine the days, weeks and months to come. This is where you can use your Self-Mastery Affirmations to optimum advantage.

Now it's time for you to write your own Self-Mastery

Affirmations. For example, if you had creativity as an impact word it could be used in an affirmation such as: "I am creatively improving my body one day at a time."

If the impact word was happiness then the affirmation could be: "I am happily drinking water to stimulate my body to be a fat burning machine." If the impact word was freedom then it could be: "I am freeing my mind to learn at an accelerated rate."

Now Take a Few Minutes to Do Your SELF-MASTERY

Affirmation Exercise

There's no time like the present to create your own Self-Mastery

Affirmations.

I have given you a great start by creating some affirmations for you. Each includes some typical impact words. Read through all the sample affirmations and circle the impact word that has greatest significance for you. If you have an impact word that's not listed, but that would have greater meaning for you, write it in the blank.

After you've completed all ten, choose the affirmation that has the most meaning to you. This is the affirmation you will use this week. Next week choose another affirmation, and then another the following week, and so on. After that, you can create your own affirmations or use any of the ten examples again. When you have determined the affirmation you want to use for the week, write it on the 3x5 card. Carry the card with you during the day and read the affirmation at least ten times a day.

Well, even though the brain and mind make up an incredibly complex system, getting it all to work for you is really quite simple, once you know how.

As you state the affirmation, imagine how you will take it with you out into the world. These affirmations can be there for you whenever a challenge or opportunity arises. Start by thinking of three places where you're going to use your affirmation. It could be when you turn on a light switch and the inner light of awareness comes on and reminds you that you are mastering life. It could happen when you turn on the ignition of your car and you ignite an affirmation to start running in your life. It could happen when you open the refrigerator door, and you remember that you are opening your mind to choices . . . and you choose to use Self-Mastery Affirmations to help you make positive changes and accomplish your loftiest goals.

Sample Affirmations

1. I am _____ improving my body each day.
   (joyfully, successfully, meaningfully, creatively, passionately)
2. I am _____ eating less, whether dining in or out. (enjoying, easily, successfully, effortlessly, simply)

3. I am really proud of myself for _____ taking the time to exercise.
   (successfully, easily, freely, happily, creatively)

4. I am _____ realizing my weight-loss goals each day. (easily, successfully, wisely, passionately, enthusiastically)

5. I am calm, relaxed and _____ as I make healthy food choices and lose weight.
   (successful, positive, creative, happy, free)

6. I am_____ drinking water to stimulate my body to be a fat burning machine.
   (easily, freely, triumphantly, confidently, joyfully)

7. I am _____ eating only those foods which are beneficial to me.
   (gladly, easily, wisely, enthusiastically, confidently)

8. I am gaining _____ everyday as I lose weight. (self-esteem, happiness, confi dence, satisfaction, freedom)

9. Right now and at all times I see myself as healthy, trim, and _____.
   (whole, happy, free, energized, light, successful)

10. I find it _____ to leave food on my plate at mealtimes. (simple, encouraging, wonderful, eff ortless, rewarding)

ADDITIONAL

RESOURCES

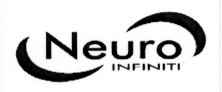

The **NeuroInfiniti** Stress Response Evaluation is an effective and accurate method of measuring your physiological stress response. It is a 12 minute computerized test, which is a totally non-invasive exam using an instrument found in research facilities around the world. Sensors are attached to your skin in such areas as your shoulder muscles, the top of your head, your forearms, and your hands. There are no needles or any form of skin penetration. From this computerized test, we can compare your neurological response and recovery to stress challenges.

For more information or to find a **NeuroInfiniti** practitioner in your area, you can contact the author at:

Richard G. Barwell, DC
NeuroInfiniti
#503 - 188 Pinellas Lane,
Cocoa Beach, Florida 32931
Phone: 321 868 5690
Email:drbarwell@neuroInifiniti.com
Website: www.NeuroInfiniti.com

Dr. Patrick Porter's
Stress-Free Lifestyle Series

Stress is the most pervasive malady of our time. The effects on our

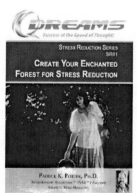

health, productivity and quality of life are more devastating than most people care to admit. Luckily, you've just found the solution! CVR can help you see yourself as the healthy, happy, optimistic person you'd prefer to be. With this new image, your fears and frustrations fade away, your anxiety vanishes, and you no longer let small things stress you.

Create Your Enchanted Forest for Stress Reduction

Follow along as Dr. Patrick Porter guides you through your personal enchanted forest—a quiet, serene place where you have nothing to do but relax. Your other-than-conscious mind will massage away all tension, allowing you to release all negative thoughts and feelings. You'll return from your magical forest filled with positive feelings, able to enjoy and express your true inner peace.

Create Your Mountaintop Retreat for Stress Reduction

Say goodbye to all stress and confusion as you take a trip to this breathtaking mountaintop retreat. When you listen to this restful process, using your mind to relax your body will become as comfortable and automatic as breathing. The stress, strain and confusion of everyday life will melt away as you awake refreshed, revitalized and renewed!

A Complete List of
Stress-Free Titles
and full descriptions
can be found at
www.brainfitnessni.com

Dr. Patrick Porter's
Vibrant Health Series

Of all the cells in your body, more than 50,000 will die and be replaced with new cells, all in the time it took you to read this sentence! Your body is the vehicle you have been given for the journey of your life. How you treat your body determines how it will treat you. Taking good care of your body will go a long way in ensuring that your life is active, happy, and full of positive experiences. Dr. Patrick Porter will show you how, by using creative visualization and relaxation (CVR), you can recharge and energize your body, mind, and spirit. This series is for people who are looking for more than good health; it's for those who will settle for nothing less than vibrant health!

Staying Focused in the Present
Your emotions can either help your body stay healthy, or they can be the cause of disease. Negative feelings such as regret, worry, or anxiety about an upcoming event not only wastes your precious life, but also adds stress to the body, which makes you more susceptible to disease. In this CVR process, Dr. Porter will help you stay present and focused on the beauty of each moment and the gift each minute offers you.

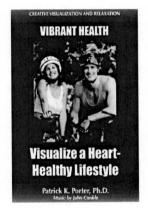

Visualize a Heart-Healthy Lifestyle
Heart disease is not a male issue alone; it is the top killer of American women. To protect your heart, you need a plan that includes movement, a healthy diet, and a positive mental attitude. You use an average of forty-three muscles to frown and only seventeen muscles to smile. You'll find smiling even easier now that you are taking an active roll in protecting the health of your heart. During this CVR session, Dr. Porter will show you how to celebrate the energy, passion, and power that are your birthright.

Check Out The Complete
Vibrant Health Series

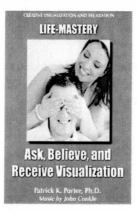

Dr. Patrick Porter's
Wealth Consciousness Series

Inspired by the principles of Napoleon Hill's Think and Grow Rich

Start Each Day with Purpose and Passion

Napoleon Hill understood that people don't plan to fail; they fail to plan. Successful people know where they are going before they start and move forward on their own initiative. They have the power of intention, or what Napoleon Hill called "mind energy," on their side. Dr. Patrick Porter (PhD) will guide you in using this power of intention to focus your imagination on the success and prosperity you desire.

Commit to a Life Spent with Like-Minded People

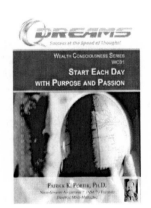

Together with Dr. Patrick Porter, you will use the power of intention to draw to yourself mastermind alliances that will support your dream. You will visualize setting up and using these mastermind alliances to help you attract goal-oriented people and create your success environment.

Trust the Power of Infinite Intelligence

Do you sometimes feel as though negative thoughts and fear of poverty have control over you? During this CVR session, Dr. Porter will guide you through the principle of applied faith. All conditions are the offspring of thought, and you find it natural to visualize and realize the thoughts and actions that bring wealth and riches into your life.

Check Out The Complete
Wealth Consciousness Series

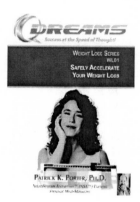

at www.brainfitnessni.com
Dr. Patrick Porter's
Accelerated Learning Series

Whether you are an honor student or just having difficulty taking a test, this breakthrough learning system will help you overcome learning challenges and accelerate your current skill level. Imagine doubling your reading speed while improving your memory. Sit back, relax and allow your mind to organize your life, while you build your self-confidence and earn better grades with the our complete learning system.

Setting Goals for Learning Success
Dr. Porter's Pikeville College study proved that the more successful students are those who have an outcome or ultimate goal in mind. With this module you will learn the secrets of goal setting, experience a boost in motivation, and see your self-confidence in the classroom soar.

Being an Optimistic Thinker
Henry Ford once said, "Whether you think you can, or you think you can't, you are right." It all starts with attitude. You will be guided into the creative state, where you'll discover ways of breaking through to your optimistic mind that will help you to think, act and respond with a positive nature even during your most difficult classes or around challenging people.

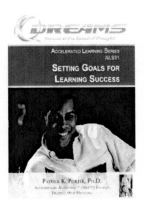

Six Steps to Using Your Perfect Memory
Harness the natural byproduct of relaxing your mind by using the six steps that activate a perfect memory. You will discover creative ways to access and recall the information you need as you need it! Best of all, you will have this ability the rest of your life.

Check Out The Complete
Accelerated Learning Series
at **www.brainfitnessni.com**

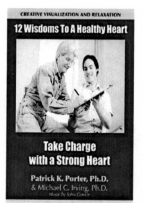

Dr. Patrick Porter's
Freedom From Addiction Series

Addiction comes in many forms, but the underlying cause remains the same. For every addiction there is an underlying positive intention that the mind is trying to fulfill. Now you can use the power of your mind—through creative visualization and relaxation (CVR)—to find more appropriate ways to satisfy that positive intention without the destructive behaviors of the past. Dr. Patrick Porter's groundbreaking CVR program for overcoming addiction can work for just about any addiction including the following:

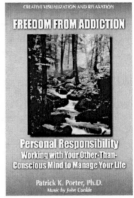

Alcoholism
Anorexia & Bulimia
Codependency
Gambling
Marijuana
Narcotics
Prescription Drugs
Overeating
Overspending
Pornography
Self-Injury
Sexual Promiscuity

Personal Responsibility —Working With Your Other-Than-Conscious Mind to Manage Your Life
Most people who struggle with addictions have, in reality, simply lost their power of choice. Dr. Patrick Porter (PhD) will help you discover why trying to force a change with willpower only perpetuates the problem and how visualization is what will lead you to realization and freedom. You will discover how, by tapping into the power of your mind, you can rebuild your confidence (even in uncertain times) and bring into your consciousness (with sufficient force) the appropriate memories and choices that will lead you to living an addiction-free life—which is your birthright.

Check Out The Complete
Freedom From Addiction Series
at **www.brainfitnessni.com**

Dr. Patrick Porter's
Coping with Cancer Series

Being diagnosed with cancer is in itself a stressful event—so stressful it can suppress your immune system and worsen the side-effects of treatment. Fortunately, through guided relaxation, you can let go

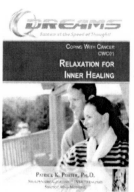

of your fear and anxiety, and take charge of your recovery. Creative visualization can help you regain an optimistic attitude, spark your immune system, and maximize your medical treatment. If you are ready to join the ranks of people who have discovered the mind/body connection and its healing potential, then the Coping with Cancer Series is definitely for you!

Relaxation For Inner Healing

For some people, relaxing while facing a serious illness may seem like an impossible task. In this first session, you will begin by simply clearing your mind of all negative or fear-based thoughts concerning your condition. At the same time, you will learn to allow the natural healing power of your body to take over. The benefits from relaxation are immeasurable when it comes to fighting cancer.

Rejuvenate Your Body Through Deep Delta Sleep

During cancer recovery, many people have difficulty falling asleep or they may awaken in the middle of the night and struggle to get back to sleep. Your body naturally recharges and rejuvenates during sleep, which means a good night's rest is key to your recovery. This imagery will show you new ways to get maximum benefit from sleep.

Check Out The Complete
Coping With Cancer Series
at www.brainfitnessni.com

Dr. Patrick Porter's
SportZone™ Series

Success in sports is about being the best you can be, and visualization plays a key role in getting there. Why is visualization so important? Because you get what you rehearse in life, but that's not always what you want or intend. This is especially true when you are facing the pressures of athletics. The SportZone program is designed to help you tap into the mind's potential and make your sport of choice fun and enjoyable while taking your game to the next level. Visualization for sports performance is nothing new to top competitors—athletes from Tiger Woods to diver Greg Louganis and a variety of Olympians have used visualization to bring about optimal performance, overcome self-doubt, and give themselves a seemingly unfair advantage over their competition. Now the SportZone series can work for any athlete, from junior competitors to weekend enthusiasts. Yes, you can get more out of your sport and, in the process, get more out of life.

Using the "Zone" in Your Sport
When competitive athletes slip into their "zone" everything seems to work just right. Dr. Patrick Porter will help you get to that place where everything comes together. With this process you'll learn to put yourself into a state of "flow," your own personal "zone," so you can stay on top of your game. The "zone" is as easy to access as a deep breath once you have mastered the mental keys.

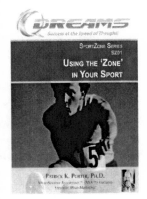

Control Your Emotions and Master Your Sport
It has been said that he or she who angers you conquers you; this is true even if the person who angers you is you! With this process you will learn a powerful self-visualization technique for keeping your emotions under control. With this easy technique you will no longer be giving away your power to others and will stop letting anger and frustration get the better of you.

Check Out The Complete
SportZone Series
at www.brainfitnessni.com

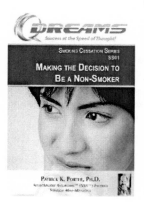

Dr. Patrick Porter's
Mental Coaching for Golf Series

Efficient golfers know how to relax and let their minds take over. Now, thanks to these creative visualization and relaxation (CVR) processes, you'll learn to see yourself as a calm, confident golfer. You deserve to take pleasure in your time on the course. Thanks to CVR, you'll finally be able to let go of frustration and focus on every stroke—meaning you'll not only play better, but you'll also enjoy the game more than ever!

Optimize the Risk Zone for Golf
You've never experienced a practice session like this one! Follow along with Dr. Patrick Porter as he guides you onto the driving range in your mind. Once there, you'll practice each swing, letting go of negative thoughts and allowing the clubs to do what they were designed to do—send the ball straight to the target.

Develop the Attitude of a Champion
Champions understand that good outcomes come from good shots. With this dynamic process, you'll find it easy to think positive thoughts and accept each shot as it comes. You'll no longer spend time feeling distracted, over-analyzing your game, blaming the conditions of the course, or getting angry over a bad lie.

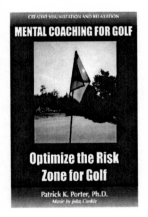

Concentration:
Your Key To Consistency
Most golf professionals consider concentration to be the key to playing golf...but almost no one teaches it. In this energizing process by Dr. Patrick Porter, he'll teach you to achieve the concentration you need simply by sitting back, relaxing, and letting go of all stress and confusion.

Check Out The Complete
Mental Coaching for Golf Series
at **www.brainfitnessni.com**

Dr. Patrick Porter's
Enlightened Children's Series

Seven-year-old Marina Mulac and five-year-old Morgan Mulac, who have come to be known as the world's youngest marketers, were the

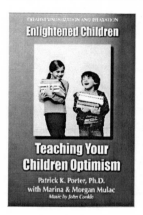

inspiration behind this Enlightened Children's Series. When they met Dr. Patrick Porter, they had one question for him: Why had he created so many great visualizations for grown ups and nothing for kids?

Dr. Porter told the two little entrepreneurs that if they put on their thinking caps and helped him design a program for kids, together they could help children from around the globe to use their imaginative minds to become better people and help improve the world. Together, Marina, Morgan, and Dr. Patrick Porter put together this series that uses guided imagery, storytelling, and positive affirmations to help children see the world as a peaceful and harmonious place where everyone can win. If your goal is to develop a happy, healthy child of influence in our rapidly changing world, this series is a must-have for your child.

Building Optimism in Your Children

Every day your child is forming his or her view of the world based on life experiences. Now is the time to help your child build a positive outlook that will serve him or her for a lifetime. Optimists believe that people and events are inherently good and that most situations work out for the best. Dr. Porter will show your child how to see the good in every situation and how to be open to experiencing new things.

Check Out The Complete
Enlightened Children's Series
at **www.brainfitnessni.com**

Dr. Patrick Porter's
Medical Series

De-Stress and Lower Blood Pressure

The physiological benefits of deep relaxation and visualization are well documented. During this creative visualization process you will learn to achieve the relaxation response—a state known to unlock your brain's potential for de-stressing your body and returning your blood pressure to a healthy level. Known benefits of the relaxation response also include a lower respiratory rate, a slower pulse, relaxed muscles, and an increase in alpha brain wave activity—everything that makes for a healthier you!

Pre-Surgery Calm for Better Healing

For years physicians and therapist have used guided relaxation, intense concentration, and focused attention to achieve deep relaxation and heightened states of awareness prior to surgery. Now, through the science of creative visualization and relaxation (CVR), you can easily benefit from these powerful processes.

Patients using these techniques are known to have less pain, require less pain medication, and enjoy a more rapid recovery.

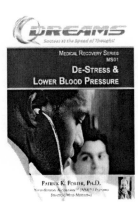

Post-Surgery Stress Relief for a Healthy Mind and Body

CVR is a relaxation technique that uses concentration and deep breathing to calm the mind and put your body in the best possible state for repair and healing. What could be easier than to sit back, relax, and let the stress of surgery and recovery melt away?

Check Out The Complete
Medical Series
at **www.brainfitnessni.com**

Dr. Patrick Porter's
Professional Airlines Blue Sky Series

The airline industry has long been considered a "glamour" industry, but those working in the business know that, once it becomes your job, you are in a constant battle to maintain the health of your body and mind. An airline professional's stress can come in many forms—from dealing with exhausting schedules and un-

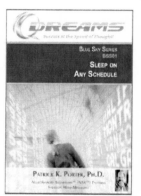

ruly passengers to the underlying fears related to travel during uncertain times. For this reason, Dr. Patrick Porter, has created the Blue Sky Series, which is designed to help airline professionals regain balance in their lives through deep relaxation and creative visualization techniques.

Sleep on Any Schedule
In the airline industry, flying across time zones, arriving late at night, and being expected to awaken early the next morning are all part of the job. While the occasional traveler is able to get over jet lag with relative ease, in the airline business, jet lag is part and parcel to a day's work. Unfortunately, this regular disruption of the sleep cycle can result in chronic fatigue, headaches, body aches, and a lowered immune system.

Clear Out Flight Noise and Return to Health
With this visualization, you will be guided through some mental balancing processes to help you deal with the impact of that constant barrage of jet engine noise. During the process you will clear your mind, reset your attention, and focus on health. You will learn to de-stress, relax, and have fun after a flight.

Check Out The Complete
Blue Sky Series
at **www.brainfitnessni.com**

Dr. Patrick Porter's
Pain-Free Lifestyle Series

Persistent pain can have a costly impact on your life. It can lead to depression, loss of appetite, irritability, anger, loss of sleep, withdrawal from social interaction, and an inability to cope. Fortunately, with creative visualization and relaxation (CVR), pain can almost always be controlled. CVR helps you eliminate pain while you relax, revitalize, and rejuvenate. You deserve to be free of your pain—and now you can be, thanks to CVR!

Tapping into a Pain-Free Lifestyle
Dr. Patrick Porter will guide you through a simple exercise to transform pain into relaxation. You'll tap into your body's innate ability to heal itself, allowing the healing process to happen while you take a relaxing mental vacation. Pain will lose all power over you as you learn to relax away your pain and enjoy your life free from discomfort.

Activate Your Mental Pharmacy
In this dynamic process, you'll unlock your body's natural pharmacy, flushing pain from your body and neutralizing all discomfort. You will so galvanize your mind's healing capacity, all you'll have to do is say the word to release pain, fear and anxiety. Most importantly, you'll have this healing power at your fingertips—when and where you need it most.

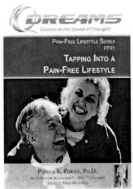

Starting the Day Pain-Free
In this motivational session, Dr. Patrick Porter will show you that living pain-free is as simple as saying, "So-Hum." Which means, transporting yourself to a pain-free state can be as easy as breathing! You'll be able to bury your pain in the past and awaken each morning pain-free.

Check Out The Complete
Pain-Free Lifestyle Series
at **www.brainfitnessni.com**

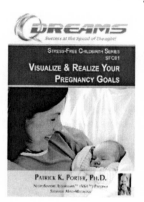

Mind-Over-Menopause Series

For many women mid-life can be a time of uncertainty and loss. For some the loss of fertility and the perceived loss of youth can cause depression and anxiety. At the same time, the body's response to the decrease in hormones can create any number of symptoms—hot flashes, night sweats, weight gain, itchy skin, mood swings, lost libido, headaches, and irregular cycles are just of few of the menopausal challenges women face. In the midst of all these changes, relationships can suffer as loved ones start to ask, "What happened to the caring, loving woman we once knew?" Now you can reclaim that woman, along with all the strength, confidence, and wisdom you gained in the first half of your life. This series takes you way beyond mind over matter—it's mind over menopause!

Balance Your Mood,
Balance Your Life
With this session you will use creative visualization and relaxation to help balance your mood, harness positive mental energy, and use your innate creative power to produce much-needed balance in your life during this time of change and uncertainty. You will stop focusing on what you've lost, and discover all that you've gained!

Creating Harmony
With the Cycles of Life
Using your mind you will activate the powerful calming effects produced by your own brain chemistry.

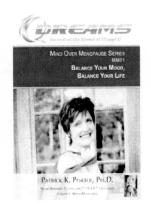

Mental Skills to Help You Master Menopause
With this creative visualization and relaxation process, you will be given time to plan your life from a new perspective. You will learn to view menopause as a rite of passage—one that gives you confidence and inner worth. With new ways to handle situations at work, and with family and friends, you'll discover that mid-life can bring forth a whole new you that's been there all along just waiting to blossom!

Check Out The Complete
Mind-Over-Menopause Series
at **www.brainfitnessni.com**

Welcome to The Gift of Love Project

The Gift of Love is a poetic writing that has its own beauty … and upon further examination, it may lead one to a contemplative process, creating balance and harmony in one's everyday life. Over time, this process can also create subtle positive change in the recipient of **The Gift**.

My guidance leads me to distribute this writing to one billion people within the next two years. Hopefully, many people will be led to practice the contemplative process. If **The Gift of Love** resonates with you, please share it with others. As we gather and hold the **power of love** in our consciousness, we will dramatically reduce the level of anger, fear, and hatred on our planet today. -- Jerry DeShazo

The Gift of Love

I Agree Today
To Be The Gift of Love.

I Agree to Feel Deeply
Love for Others
Independent of Anything
They Are Expressing,
Saying, Doing, or Being.

I Agree to Allow Love
As I Know It
To Embrace My Whole Body
And Then to Just Send It
To Them Silently and Secretly.

I Agree to Feel it, Accept it, Breathe It
Into Every Cell of My Body on Each In-Breath
And On Each Out-Breath
Exhale Any Feeling Unlike Love.

I Will Repeat This Breathing Process Multiple Times
Until I Feel it Fully and Completely
Then Consciously Amplify In Me
The Feeling of Love and Project It to Others
As The Gift of Love.

This is My Secret Agreement –
No One Else Is To Know it.

For more about The Gift of Love Project and to view the videos, please visit www.TheGiftofLove.com. You will also be given access to a special 9-minute Creative Visualization that will align you with the **Power of Love** and supercharge your day. Together we will change the world one person at a time.

CPSIA information can be obtained at www.ICGtesting.com
Printed in the USA
LVOW07s0012250615

443796LV00002B/6/P